Breath Sounds

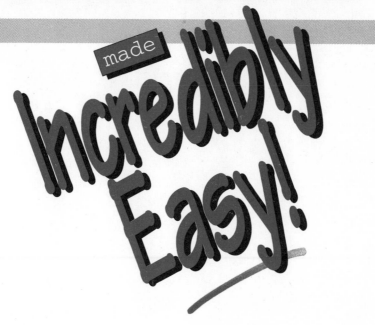

made
Incredibly
Easy!

Breath Sounds

made Incredibly Easy!®

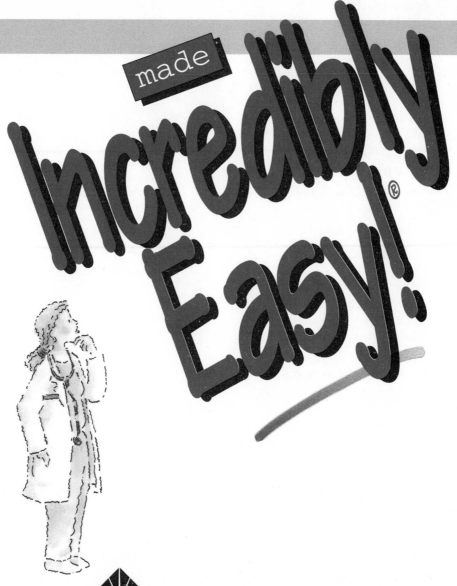

LIPPINCOTT WILLIAMS & WILKINS
A **Wolters Kluwer** Company

Philadelphia • Baltimore • New York • London
Buenos Aires • Hong Kong • Sydney • Tokyo

Staff

Executive Publisher
Judith A. Schilling McCann, RN, MSN

Editorial Director
David Moreau

Clinical Director
Joan M. Robinson, RN, MSN

Senior Art Director
Arlene Putterman

Art Director
Mary Ludwicki

Electronic Project Manager
John Macalino

Editorial Project Manager
Jaime Stockslager Buss

Clinical Project Manager
Roseanne Hanlon Rafter, RN, MSN, CS

Editors
Dave Beverage, Laura Bruck, Diane Labus,
Julie Munden, Liz Schaeffer, Gale Thompson

Clinical Editor
Tamara M. Kear, RN, MSN, CNN

Copy Editors
Kimberly Bilotta (supervisor), Scotti Cohn, Shana
Harrington, Dorothy P. Terry, Pamela Wingrod

Designer
Lynn Foulk

Illustrator
Bot Roda

Digital Composition Services
Diane Paluba (manager), Joyce Rossi Biletz,
Richard Eng

Manufacturing
Patricia K. Dorshaw (director), Beth J. Welsh

Editorial Assistants
Megan L. Aldinger, Tara L. Carter-Bell,
Linda K. Ruhf

Indexer
Barbara Hodgson

BRTHSIE010904 — 040207

Library of Congress Cataloging-in-Publication Data
Breath sounds made incredibly easy!
    p. ; cm.
    Includes bibliographical references and index.
    1. Auscultation. 2. Respiratory organs — Sounds.
    3. Respiratory organs — Pathophysiology. 4. Respiratory
    organs — Diseases — Diagnosis. I. Lippincott Williams &
    Wilkins.
    [DNLM: 1. Respiratory Sounds. WF 102 B8284 2005]
RC734.A94B74 2005
616.07'544—dc22
ISBN13: 978-1-58255-354-2
ISBN 1-58255-354-8 (alk. paper)   2004011279

Contents

Contributors and consultants

Janice Hausauer, RN, MS, FNP
Adjunct Assistant Professor
Montana State University College of Nursing
Bozeman

Nancy Haynes, RN, MN, CCRN
Assistant Professor
Saint Luke's College
Kansas City, Mo.

Foreword

The ability to accurately collect and interpret clinical assessment data is the cornerstone of effective nursing care. Even with today's technological advances in health care, accurate data collection and interpretation are irreplaceable. However, attaining expert assessment skills doesn't happen overnight. To build confidence in these skills, the nurse must have a working knowledge of anatomy and physiology and use a straightforward examination approach. Such confidence not only improves patient care but also enhances professional satisfaction.

Breath Sounds Made Incredibly Easy covers the key information that will help the novice and the experienced nurse gain competence in assessing the respiratory system. The text begins with an overview of important anatomy and physiology concepts. Numerous illustrations enhance understanding of the text. The subsequent clinical assessment chapter includes information on obtaining a patient's health history, which helps refine interview skills specific to respiratory conditions. The essential steps of inspection, percussion, and palpation are also presented, providing the reader with the information needed to perform a thorough and clinically useful respiratory system examination.

The auscultation content is organized so that the reader becomes familiar with how normal breath sounds are produced, what they sound like, and how these sounds are classified. Common abnormal breath sounds are also discussed. These sounds are correlated with common pathophysiological conditions, thus linking the book's content to ambulatory care and bedside practice. For most of the breath sounds covered, you'll find illustrations that clarify the physiology and guide your auscultation.

Breath Sounds Made Incredibly Easy concludes with an excellent and easy-to-follow overview of respiratory disorders, ranging from common chronic conditions, such as chronic obstructive pulmonary disease, to life-threatening disorders, such as acute respiratory failure. Each condition is broken down into essential, need-to-know components: causes, signs and symptoms, and interventions. Each chapter closes with a *Quick quiz* that helps to assess the reader's understanding of key concepts.

Several features of *Breath Sounds Made Incredibly Easy* allow the nurse to rapidly incorporate new knowledge into clinical practice. Throughout the text, you'll encounter:

Breathe easy — simplifies difficult concepts using illustrations and clear, simple explanations

Inspired work — offers tips for honing your auscultation skills, including the proper way to listen for particular sounds

Memory jogger — reinforces important information and offers you an easy way to remember it

Ages and stages — highlights important age-related differences in auscultation findings.

Because a large part of respiratory system assessment relies on interpreting auscultatory findings, you'll also find an accompanying CD in the back of *Breath Sounds Made Incredibly Easy.* Cues to the audio are embedded in the text, but the CD can also be reviewed independently. This convenient feature makes *Breath Sounds Made Incredibly Easy* suitable for individual or group study.

The time invested in reading *Breath Sounds Made Incredibly Easy* and listening to the accompanying CD will result in enhanced knowledge and refined auscultation skills. When you apply this knowledge and these skills, you'll be amazed by what you learn from a well-conducted examination. So, grab your stethoscope and jump right in. You'll be glad you did!

Lynda A. Mackin, APRN,BC, MS, CNS, ANP
Assistant Clinical Professor
School of Nursing
University of California, San Francisco

① Anatomy and physiology

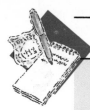

Just the facts

In this chapter, you'll learn:

♦ structures of the respiratory system and their functions

♦ principles of inspiration and expiration

♦ process for gas exchange in the alveoli

♦ impact of nervous, musculoskeletal, and pulmonary disorders on breathing

♦ role of the lungs in acid-base balance.

The respiratory system at a glance

The respiratory system consists of the upper respiratory tract, lower respiratory tract (including the lungs), and thoracic cavity. In addition to maintaining the exchange of oxygen and carbon dioxide in the lungs and tissues, the respiratory system also helps regulate the body's acid-base balance.

Upper respiratory tract

The upper respiratory tract consists primarily of the mouth, nose, pharynx, nasopharynx, oropharynx, laryngopharynx, and larynx. These structures warm and humidify inspired air. They're also responsible for taste, smell, and the chewing and swallowing of food. (See *Picturing the respiratory system*, page 2.)

Your upper respiratory tract helps you enjoy every aspect of a delicious meal.

Picturing the respiratory system

The illustration below can help you visualize the structures of the respiratory system.

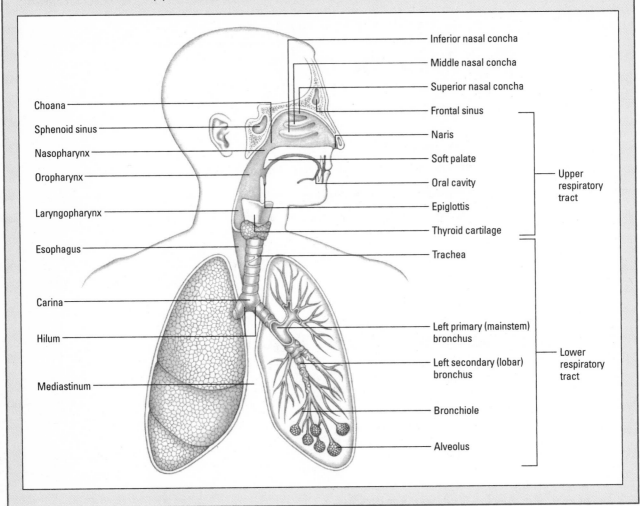

Choana	Inferior nasal concha
Sphenoid sinus	Middle nasal concha
Nasopharynx	Superior nasal concha
Oropharynx	Frontal sinus
Laryngopharynx	Naris
Esophagus	Soft palate
Carina	Oral cavity
Hilum	Epiglottis
Mediastinum	Thyroid cartilage
	Trachea

Upper respiratory tract

Left primary (mainstem) bronchus

Left secondary (lobar) bronchus

Bronchiole

Alveolus

Lower respiratory tract

Nose and nasal passages

Air enters the body through the nares (nostrils). In the nares, small hairs known as *vibrissae* filter out dust and large foreign particles. Air then passes into the two nasal passages, which are separated by the septum. Cartilage forms the anterior walls of the nasal passages; bony structures (known as *turbinates*, or *conchae*) form the posterior walls. The superior, middle, and inferior turbinates are separated by grooves, called *meatus*.

Just passing through

The curved bony turbinates and their mucosal covering ease breathing by warming, filtering, and humidifying inhaled air before it passes into the nasopharynx. Their mucus layer also traps finer foreign particles, which the cilia carry to the pharynx to be swallowed.

Sinus language

The sinuses serve as resonators for sound production and provide mucus. Four pairs of paranasal sinuses open into the internal nose:
• The maxillary sinuses are located on the cheeks below the eyes.
• The frontal sinuses are located above the eyebrows.
• The ethmoidal and sphenoidal sinuses are located behind the eyes and nose in the head.

Pharynx and nasopharynx

The pharynx is composed of striated muscle and lined with a mucous membrane. It serves as a passageway for air entering from the nose. Air passes from the nasal cavity into the muscular nasopharynx through the choanae, a pair of posterior openings in the nasal cavity that remain constantly open.

Oropharynx and laryngopharynx

The oropharynx is the posterior wall of the mouth. It connects the nasopharynx and the laryngopharynx. The laryngopharynx extends to the esophagus and larynx.

Larynx

The larynx connects the pharynx with the trachea. It also contains the vocal cords. Muscles and cartilage form the walls of the larynx, including the large, shield-shaped thyroid cartilage situated just under the jaw line.

Listen up! The vocal cords are located in the larynx.

Lower respiratory tract

The lower respiratory tract consists of the trachea, bronchi, and lungs. Functionally, the lower tract is subdivided into the conducting airways and the acinus. The acinus serves as the area of gas exchange. A mucous membrane that contains hairlike cilia lines the lower tract. Cilia constantly clean the tract and carry foreign matter upward for swallowing or expectoration.

> I like things nice and tidy. Cilia help keep the airways clean.

Conducting airways

The conducting airways, which contain the trachea and bronchi, help facilitate gas exchange.

Trachea

The trachea extends from the cricoid cartilage at the top to the carina (also called the *tracheal bifurcation*). The carina is a ridge-shaped structure at the level of the sixth or seventh thoracic vertebra. C-shaped cartilage rings reinforce and protect the trachea to prevent it from collapsing.

Bronchi

The primary bronchi begin at the carina. The left mainstem bronchus delivers air to the left lung. The right mainstem bronchus—shorter, wider, and more vertical than the left—supplies air to the right lung.

Divide and conquer

The mainstem bronchi divide into five lobar bronchi (secondary bronchi). Along with blood vessels, nerves, and lymphatics, the secondary bronchi enter the pleural cavities and the lungs at the hilum. Located behind the heart, the hilum is a slit on the lung's medial surface where the lungs are anchored.

Bronchi branch out

Each lobar bronchus enters a lobe in each lung. Within its lobe, each of the lobar bronchi branches into segmental bronchi (tertiary bronchi). The segments continue to branch into smaller and smaller bronchi, finally branching into bronchioles.

The larger bronchi consist of cartilage, smooth muscle, and epithelium. As the bronchi become smaller, they first lose cartilage, then smooth muscle until, finally, the smallest bronchioles consist of just a single layer of epithelial cells.

Acinus

Each bronchiole includes an acinus — the chief respiratory unit for gas exchange. The acinus consists of respiratory bronchioles and alveoli. (See *Picturing the pulmonary airway*.)

Picturing the pulmonary airway

As illustrated below, each bronchiole contains terminal bronchioles and the acinus, consisting of respiratory bronchioles and alveolar sacs.

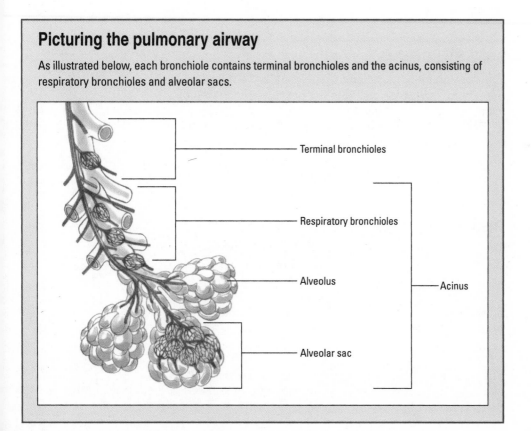

Terminal bronchioles

Respiratory bronchioles

Alveolus

Alveolar sac

Acinus

Respiratory bronchioles

Within the acinus, terminal bronchioles branch into yet smaller respiratory bronchioles. The respiratory bronchioles feed directly into alveoli at sites along their walls.

Alveolar walls contain two basic epithelial cell types:

☝   Type I cells, which are the most abundant, are thin, flat, squamous cells. Gas exchange occurs across these cells.

✌   Type II cells secrete surfactant, a substance that coats the alveolus and promotes gas exchange by lowering surface tension.

Alveoli

The respiratory bronchioles eventually become alveolar ducts, which terminate in clusters of capillary-swathed alveoli called *alveolar sacs*. Gas exchange takes place through the alveoli.

Lungs and accessory structures

The cone-shaped lungs hang suspended in the right and left pleural cavities, straddling the heart and anchored by root and pulmonary ligaments.

The right lung is shorter, broader, and larger than the left. It has three lobes and handles 55% of gas exchange. The left lung has two lobes. Each lung's concave base rests on the diaphragm; the apex extends about ½″ (1.3 cm) above the first rib.

Pleura and pleural cavities

The pleura—the serous membrane that totally encloses the lung—is composed of a visceral layer and a parietal layer. The visceral pleura hugs the entire lung surface, including the areas between the lobes. The parietal pleura lines the inner surface of the chest wall and upper surface of the diaphragm.

Serous fluid's serious functions

The pleural cavity—the tiny area between the visceral and parietal pleural layers—contains a thin film of serous fluid. This fluid has two functions:

> The word *visceral* refers to a body organ; therefore, the visceral pleura covers the lungs. The word *parietal* refers to a body cavity, so it makes sense that the parietal pleura covers the chest wall.

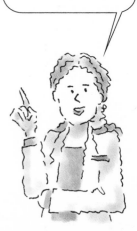

☝   It lubricates the pleural surfaces so that they slide smoothly against each other as the lungs expand and contract.

✌   It creates a bond between the layers that causes the lungs to move with the chest wall during breathing.

Thoracic cavity

The thoracic cavity is an area that's surrounded by the diaphragm (below), the scalene muscles and fasciae of the neck (above), and the ribs, intercostal muscles, vertebrae, sternum, and ligaments (around the circumference). Within the thoracic cavity are the mediastinum and the thoracic cage.

Mediastinum

The space between the lungs is called the mediastinum. It contains the:
- heart and pericardium
- thoracic aorta
- pulmonary artery and veins
- venae cavae and azygos veins
- thymus, lymph nodes, and vessels
- trachea, esophagus, and thoracic duct
- vagus, cardiac, and phrenic nerves.

Thoracic cage

Composed of bone and cartilage, the thoracic cage supports and protects the lungs, allowing them to expand and contract. The thoracic cage is divided into a posterior and an anterior portion.

Posterior thoracic cage

The vertebral column and 12 pairs of ribs comprise the posterior portion of the thoracic cage. The ribs constitute the major portion of the thoracic cage. They extend from the thoracic vertebrae toward the anterior thorax.

> The thoracic cage offers me support as well as protection, which allows me to do my job.

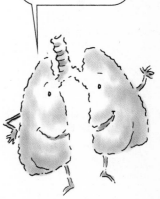

Locating lung structures in the thoracic cage

The ribs, vertebrae, and other structures of the thoracic cage act as landmarks that you can use to identify underlying structures.

From the front
• The base of each lung rests at the level of the sixth rib at the midclavicular line and the eighth rib at the midaxillary line.
• The apex of each lung extends about ¾″ to 1½″ (2 to 4 cm) above the inner aspects of the clavicles.
• The upper lobe of the right lung ends level with the fourth rib at the midclavicular line and with the fifth rib at the midaxillary line.
• The middle lobe of the right lung extends triangularly from the fourth to the sixth rib at the midclavicular line and to the fifth rib at the midaxillary line.
• Because the left lung does not have a middle lobe, the upper lobe of the left lung ends level with the fourth rib at the midclavicular line and with the fifth rib at the midaxillary line.

From the back
• The lungs extend from the cervical area to the level of the tenth thoracic vertebra (T10). On deep inspiration, the lungs may descend to T12.
• An imaginary line, stretching from the T3 level along the inferior border of the scapulae to the fifth rib at

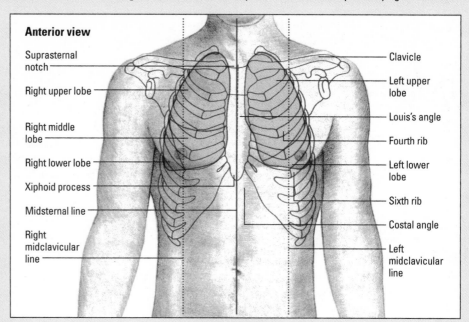

Anterior view

Suprasternal notch
Right upper lobe
Right middle lobe
Right lower lobe
Xiphoid process
Midsternal line
Right midclavicular line

Clavicle
Left upper lobe
Louis's angle
Fourth rib
Left lower lobe
Sixth rib
Costal angle
Left midclavicular line

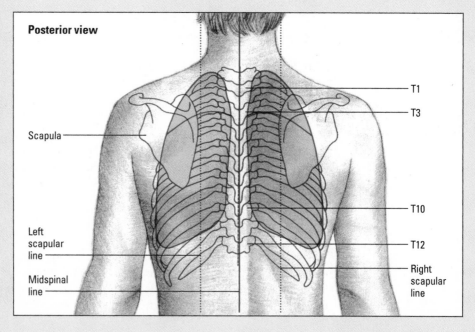

Posterior view

Scapula
Left scapular line
Midspinal line

T1
T3
T10
T12
Right scapular line

Locating lung structures in the thoracic cage *(continued)*

the midaxillary line, separates the upper lobes of both lungs.

• The upper lobes exist above T3; the lower lobes exist below T3 and extend to the level of T10.

• The diaphragm originates around the ninth or tenth rib.

From the side

• The right and left lateral rib cages cover the lobes of the right and left lungs, respectively.

• Beneath these structures, the lungs extend from just above the clavicles to the level of the eighth rib.

• The left lateral thorax allows access to two lobes; the right lateral thorax, to three lobes.

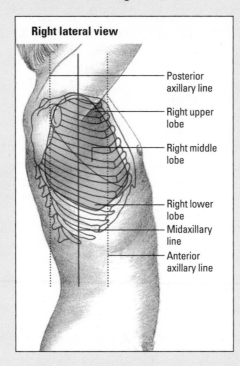

Right lateral view

Posterior axillary line

Right upper lobe

Right middle lobe

Right lower lobe

Midaxillary line

Anterior axillary line

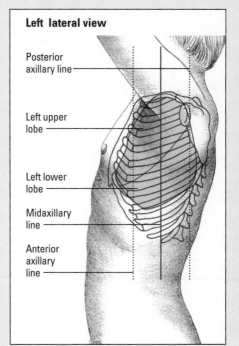

Left lateral view

Posterior axillary line

Left upper lobe

Left lower lobe

Midaxillary line

Anterior axillary line

Anterior thoracic cage

The anterior thoracic cage consists of the manubrium, sternum, xiphoid process, and ribs. It protects the mediastinal organs that lie between the right and left pleural cavities.

Counting ribs

Ribs 1 through 7 attach directly to the sternum; ribs 8 through 10 attach to the cartilage of the preceding rib. The other 2 pairs of ribs are "free-floating" — they don't attach to any part of the anterior thoracic cage. Rib 11 ends anterolaterally, and rib 12 ends laterally.

Bordering on the costal angle

The lower portion of the rib cage (costal margins) near the xiphoid process forms the borders of the costal angle — an angle of about 90 degrees in a normal person. (See *Locating lung structures in the thoracic cage*.)

It's suprasternal

Above the anterior thorax is a depression called the *suprasternal notch*. Because the rib cage doesn't cover the suprasternal notch, as it does the rest of the thorax, the trachea and aortic pulsation can be palpated here.

Inspiration and expiration

Breathing involves two actions: inspiration (an active process) and expiration (a relatively passive process). Both actions rely on respiratory muscle function and the effects of pressure differences in the lungs.

It's perfectly normal!

During normal respiration, the external intercostal muscles aid the diaphragm, the major muscle of respiration. The diaphragm descends to lengthen the chest cavity, while the external intercostal muscles (located between and along the lower borders of the ribs) contract to expand the anteroposterior diameter. This coordinated action causes inspiration. Rising of the diaphragm and relaxation of the intercostal muscles cause expiration. (See *Mechanics of respiration*.)

Forced inspiration and active expiration

During exercise, when the body needs increased oxygenation, or in certain disease states that require forced inspiration and active expiration, the accessory muscles of respiration also participate.

Forced inspiration

During forced inspiration:
• the pectoral muscles (upper chest) raise the chest to increase the anteroposterior diameter
• the sternocleidomastoid muscles (side of neck) raise the sternum
• the scalene muscles (in the neck) elevate, fix, and expand the upper chest
• the posterior trapezius muscles (upper back) raise the thoracic cage.

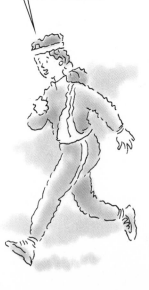

When I'm exercising, my accessory muscles of respiration kick in to make sure I get enough air.

Mechanics of respiration

The muscles of respiration help the chest cavity expand and contract. Pressure differences between atmospheric air and the lungs help produce air movement. These illustrations show the muscles that work together to allow inspiration and expiration.

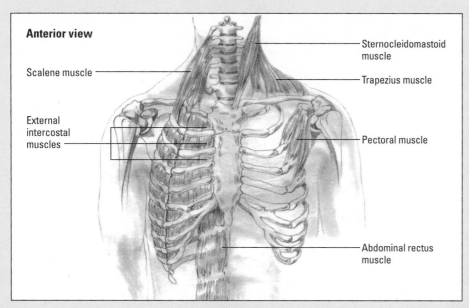

Anterior view

Scalene muscle

External intercostal muscles

Sternocleidomastoid muscle

Trapezius muscle

Pectoral muscle

Abdominal rectus muscle

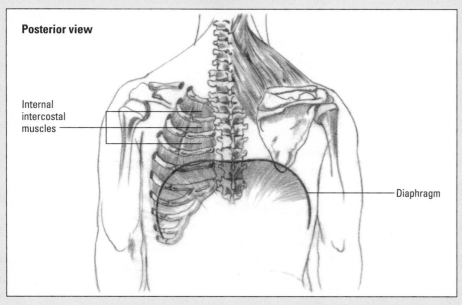

Posterior view

Internal intercostal muscles

Diaphragm

Active expiration

During active expiration, the internal intercostal muscles contract to shorten the chest's transverse diameter and the abdominal rectus muscles pull down the lower chest, thus depressing the lower ribs.

Gas station

Oxygen-depleted blood enters the lungs from the pulmonary artery of the heart's right ventricle. It then flows through the main pulmonary arteries into the smaller vessels of the pleural cavities and the main bronchi, through the arterioles and, eventually, to the capillary networks in the alveoli. In the alveoli, gas exchange — oxygen and carbon dioxide diffusion — takes place. (See *Tracing pulmonary circulation.*)

External and internal respiration

Effective respiration consists of gas exchange in the lungs, called *external respiration,* and gas exchange in the tissues, called *internal respiration.*

External respiration occurs through three processes:

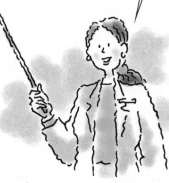

Respiration occurs internally, in the tissues, as well as externally, in the lungs.

☞   ventilation — gas distribution into and out of the pulmonary airways

✌   pulmonary perfusion — blood flow from the right side of the heart, through the pulmonary circulation, and into the left side of the heart

🖐   diffusion — gas movement through a semipermeable membrane from an area of greater concentration to one of lesser concentration.

Internal respiration occurs only through diffusion.

Ventilation

Ventilation is the distribution of gases (oxygen and carbon dioxide) into and out of the pulmonary airways. Problems within the nervous, musculoskeletal, and pulmonary systems greatly compromise breathing effectiveness.

A head game

Involuntary breathing results from stimulation of the respiratory center in the medulla and the pons of the brain.

Breathe easy

Tracing pulmonary circulation

The right and left pulmonary arteries carry deoxygenated blood from the right side of the heart to the lungs. These arteries divide into distal branches, called *arterioles,* which eventually terminate as a concentrated capillary network in the alveoli and alveolar sac, where gas exchange occurs.

Venules—the end branches of the pulmonary veins—collect oxygenated blood from the capillaries and transport it to larger vessels, which in turn lead to the pulmonary veins. The pulmonary veins enter the left side of the heart and provide oxygenated blood to the body.

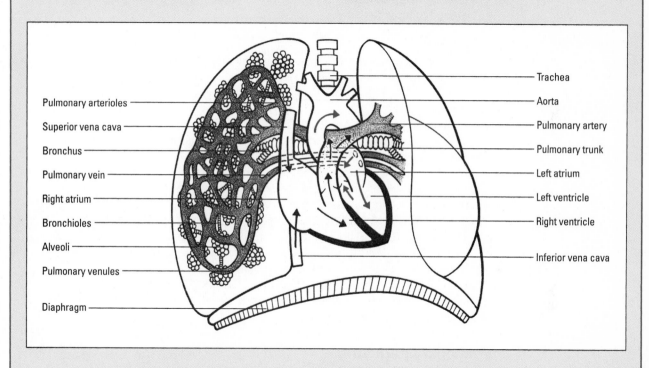

Pulmonary arterioles

Superior vena cava

Bronchus

Pulmonary vein

Right atrium

Bronchioles

Alveoli

Pulmonary venules

Diaphragm

Trachea

Aorta

Pulmonary artery

Pulmonary trunk

Left atrium

Left ventricle

Right ventricle

Inferior vena cava

The medulla controls the rate and depth of respiration; the pons moderates the rhythm of the switch from inspiration to expiration.

Under pressure

The medulla controls ventilation primarily by stimulating contraction of the diaphragm and external intercostal muscles. Because the adult thorax is flexible, contraction of the chest muscles changes its shape. In turn, this produces intrapulmonary pressure changes, triggering inspiration.

Road blocks

Many factors affect airflow distribution. These factors include:
• airflow pattern (see *Comparing airflow patterns*)
• volume and location of the functional reserve capacity (air retained in the alveoli that prevents their collapse during respiration)
• degree of intrapulmonary resistance
• presence of lung disease.

The path of least resistance

If airflow is disrupted for any reason, airflow distribution follows the path of least resistance.

Forcing the issue

Other musculoskeletal and intrapulmonary factors can affect airflow and, in turn, may affect breathing. For example, forced breathing, as in emphysema, activates accessory muscles of respiration. Using these muscles increases the workload of breathing, which requires additional oxygen and results in less efficient ventilation.

Other airflow alterations can also increase oxygen and energy demand and cause respiratory muscle fatigue. These conditions include interference with expansion of the lungs or thorax (changes in compliance) and interference with airflow in the tracheobronchial tree (changes in resistance). (See *Respiratory changes with aging.*)

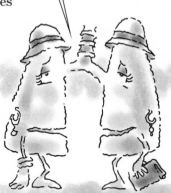

I love lots of accessories, but using my accessory muscles to breathe wears me out!

Pulmonary perfusion

Pulmonary perfusion refers to blood flow from the right side of the heart, through the pulmonary circulation, and into the left side of the heart. Perfusion aids external respiration. Normal pulmonary blood flow allows alveolar gas exchange; however, many factors may interfere with gas transport to the alveoli. Here are some examples:
• Cardiac output less than the average of 5 L/minute reduces blood flow, which decreases gas exchange.
• Elevations in pulmonary and systemic resistance also reduce blood flow.

Comparing airflow patterns

The pattern of airflow through the respiratory passages affects airway resistance.

Laminar flow

Laminar flow, a linear pattern that occurs at low flow rates, offers minimal resistance. This flow type occurs mainly in the small peripheral airways of the bronchial tree.

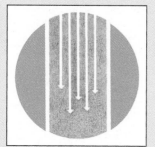

Turbulent flow

The eddying pattern of turbulent flow creates friction and increases resistance. Turbulent flow is normal in the trachea and large central bronchi. If the smaller airways become constricted or clogged with secretions, however, turbulent flow may also occur there.

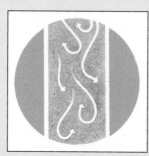

Transitional flow

A mixed pattern known as transitional flow is common at lower flow rates in the larger airways, especially where the airways narrow from obstruction, meet, or branch.

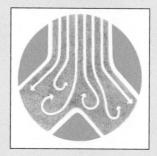

Ages and stages

Respiratory changes with aging

Aging causes decreased compliance of the lungs and chest wall. Maximal lung function decreases with age, but breathing should remain adequate. In nonsmokers, changes caused by aging don't cause clinically significant airway obstruction or dyspnea.

• Abnormal or insufficient hemoglobin picks up less oxygen for exchange.

Have gravity, will travel

Gravity can affect oxygen and carbon dioxide transport in a positive way. Gravity causes more unoxygenated blood to travel to the lower and middle lung lobes than to the upper lobes. This explains why ventilation and perfusion differ in various parts of the lungs. Areas where perfusion and ventilation are similar have what's referred to as a ventilation-perfusion match; in such areas, gas exchange is most efficient. (See *What happens in ventilation-perfusion mismatch*, page 16.)

Diffusion

In diffusion, oxygen and carbon dioxide molecules move between the alveoli and capillaries. The movement always

What happens in ventilation-perfusion mismatch

Ideally, the amount of air in the alveoli (a reflection of ventilation) should match the amount of blood in the capillaries (a reflection of perfusion). This allows gas exchange to proceed smoothly.

In actuality, the ventilation-perfusion ($\dot{V}/\dot{Q}$) ratio is unequal: The alveoli receive air at a rate of approximately 4 L/minute, while the capillaries supply blood at a rate of about 5 L/minute. This creates a $\dot{V}/\dot{Q}$ mismatch of 4:5, or 0.8.

Normal
In the normal lung, ventilation closely matches perfusion.

Shunt
Perfusion without ventilation usually results from airway obstruction, particularly that caused by acute diseases, such as atelectasis and pneumonia.

Dead-space ventilation
Normal ventilation without perfusion usually results from a perfusion defect such as pulmonary embolism.

Silent unit
Absence of ventilation and perfusion usually stems from multiple causes, such as pulmonary embolism with resultant acute respiratory distress syndrome and emphysema.

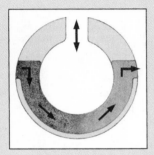
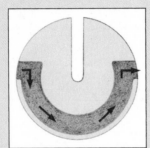
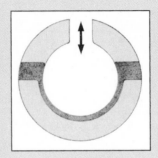
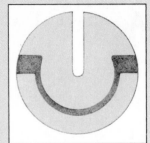

proceeds from an area of greater concentration to one of lesser concentration. In the process, oxygen moves across the alveolar and capillary membranes, dissolves in the plasma, and then passes through the red blood cell (RBC) membrane. Carbon dioxide moves in the opposite direction.

Spaces in between

For successful diffusion, the epithelial membranes lining the alveoli and capillaries must be intact. Both the alveolar epithelium and the capillary endothelium are composed of a single layer of cells. Between these layers are tiny interstitial spaces filled with elastin and collagen.

A binding proposition

Normally, oxygen and carbon dioxide move easily through all of these layers. Oxygen moves from the alveoli into the bloodstream. Once there, most of it binds with hemoglobin to form oxyhemoglobin; however, a small portion dissolves in plasma. (The portion of oxygen that dissolves in plasma can be measured as the partial pressure of oxygen in arterial blood, or PaO_2.) When oxygen binds with hemoglobin, it displaces carbon dioxide (the by-product of metabolism). The carbon dioxide diffuses from the RBCs into the blood, where it travels to the alveoli.

A working relationship

After oxygen binds to hemoglobin, the RBCs travel to the tissues. Through cellular diffusion, the RBCs release oxygen and absorb carbon dioxide. The RBCs then transport the carbon dioxide back to the lungs for removal during expiration. This is known as internal respiration. (See *Exchanging gases*, page 18.)

Acid-base balance

Oxygen taken up in the lungs is transported to the tissues by the circulatory system, which exchanges it for carbon dioxide produced by metabolism in body cells. Because carbon dioxide is more soluble than oxygen, it dissolves in the blood. In the blood, most of the carbon dioxide forms bicarbonate (base) and smaller amounts form carbonic acid (acid).

The lungs control bicarbonate levels by converting bicarbonate to carbon dioxide and water for excretion. In response to signals from the medulla, the lungs can change the rate and depth of breathing. This change allows for adjustments in the amount of carbon dioxide loss, which help to maintain acid-base balance.

Just blow it off

For example, in metabolic acidosis (a condition resulting from excess acid retention or excess bicarbonate loss), the lungs increase the rate and depth of ventilation to eliminate excess carbon dioxide, thus reducing carbonic acid levels. In metabolic alkalosis (a condition resulting from excess bicarbonate retention), the rate and depth of ventilation decrease so

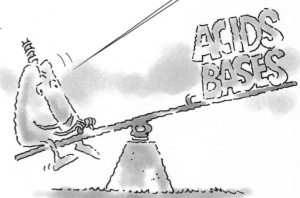

The lungs help keep the body's acid-base system in balance.

Breathe easy

Exchanging gases

Gas exchange occurs very rapidly in the millions of tiny, thin-membraned alveoli within the respiratory units. Inside these air sacs, oxygen from inhaled air diffuses into the blood while carbon dioxide diffuses from the blood into the air and is exhaled. Blood then circulates throughout the body, delivering oxygen and picking up carbon dioxide. Finally, the blood returns to the lungs to be oxygenated again.

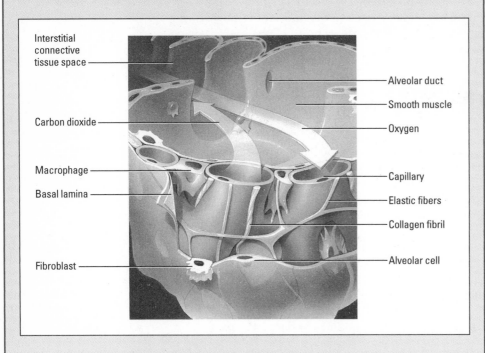

Interstitial connective tissue space

Carbon dioxide

Macrophage

Basal lamina

Fibroblast

Alveolar duct

Smooth muscle

Oxygen

Capillary

Elastic fibers

Collagen fibril

Alveolar cell

that carbon dioxide can be retained; this increases carbonic acid levels.

Uneven exchange

When the lungs don't function properly, an acid-base imbalance results. For example, they can cause respiratory acidosis through hypoventilation (reduced rate and depth of ventilation), which leads to carbon dioxide retention. They can also cause respiratory alkalosis through hyperventilation (increased rate and depth of ventilation), which leads to carbon dioxide elimination.

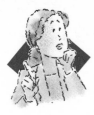

Quick quiz

1. Gas exchange takes place through the:
    A.   sinuses and pharynx.
    B.   conchae.
    C.   alveoli.
    D.   trachea.

Answer: C. Gas exchange takes place through the alveoli.

2. The space between the lungs is known as the:
    A.   thoracic cage.
    B.   mediastinum.
    C.   pleura.
    D.   hilum.

Answer: B. The space between the lungs is known as the mediastinum.

3. Involuntary breathing results from stimulation of:
    A.   the pulmonary arterioles.
    B.   the bronchioles.
    C.   the alveolar capillary network.
    D.   the respiratory center in the medulla and pons of the brain.

Answer: D. Involuntary breathing results from stimulation of the respiratory center in the medulla and pons of the brain.

4. The rate and depth of ventilation decrease so that carbon dioxide can be retained in:
    A.   metabolic acidosis.
    B.   metabolic alkalosis.
    C.   ventilation-perfusion mismatch.
    D.   conditions with excess bicarbonate loss.

Answer: B. The rate and depth of ventilation decrease so that carbon dioxide can be retained in metabolic alkalosis.

5. Above the anterior thorax is a depression known as:
    A.   the suprasternal notch.
    B.   the xiphoid process.
    C.   the scapula.
    D.   Louis's angle.

Answer: A. The suprasternal notch is a depression located above the anterior thorax. Because the rib cage doesn't cover this notch, the tracheal and aortic pulsations can be palpated here.

6. Gas exchange that occurs in the tissues is called:
   A. external respiration.
   B. ventilation.
   C. internal respiration.
   D. pulmonary perfusion.

Answer: C. Internal respiration is gas exchange that occurs in the tissues. External respiration is gas exchange that occurs in the lungs through the processes of ventilation, pulmonary perfusion, and diffusion.

Scoring

☆☆☆ If you answered all six questions correctly, take a deep breath! You've got a good grasp on respiratory system anatomy and physiology.

☆☆ If you answered four or five questions correctly, way to go! You're breezing through these systems like a whirlwind.

☆ If you answered fewer than four questions correctly, get inspired! There are plenty of *Quick quizzes* to go!

Assessment

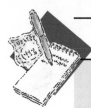

Just the facts

In this chapter, you'll learn:
♦ ways to obtain a health history
♦ techniques for assessing the respiratory system
♦ characteristics of normal breath sounds.

Respiratory assessment at a glance

Because the body depends on the respiratory system to survive, respiratory assessment is a critical nursing responsibility. Performing a comprehensive respiratory assessment requires knowledge of the respiratory system, accurate data collection, and recognition of abnormalities. A detailed health history and systematic physical examination can help you identify respiratory changes in the patient.

Obtaining a health history

The information you gain from the patient's medical history helps you understand his present symptoms. When obtaining a health history, focus your questioning on complaints of shortness of breath, cough, sputum production, wheezing, and chest pain. (See *Breathtaking facts*, page 22.)

You take my breath away

Begin by asking the patient about any complaints of dyspnea (shortness of breath). Ask him to rate his usual level

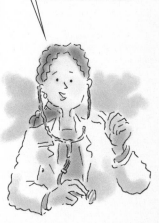

The body depends on the respiratory system to survive. That makes respiratory assessment a critical nursing responsibility.

Breathtaking facts

A quick review of your patient's health history can reveal a lot about his current problem.

Cough drops
Coughing clears unwanted material from the tracheobronchial tree. Also, sputum from the bronchial tubes traps foreign matter and protects the lungs from damage.

Pain sites
The lungs don't contain pain receptors; however, chest pain may be caused by inflammation of the pleura or the costochondral joints at the midclavicular line or at the edge of the sternum.

How much oxygen?
Patients with chronically high partial pressure of arterial carbon dioxide ($Paco_2$), such as those with chronic obstructive pulmonary disease or a neuromuscular disease, may be stimulated to breathe by a low oxygen level (the hypoxic drive) rather than by a slightly high $Paco_2$ level, as is normal. For such patients, supplemental oxygen therapy should be provided cautiously because it may depress the stimulus to breathe, further increasing $Paco_2$.

Grading dyspnea

To assess dyspnea as objectively as possible, ask your patient to briefly describe how various activities affect his breathing. Then document his response using this grading system.

Grade 0: Not troubled by breathlessness except with strenuous exercise
Grade 1: Troubled by shortness of breath when hurrying on a level path or walking up a slight hill
Grade 2: Walks more slowly on a level path because of breathlessness than people of the same age or has to stop to breathe when walking on a level path at his own pace
Grade 3: Stops to breathe after walking about 100 yards (91 m) on a level path
Grade 4: Too breathless to leave the house or breathless when dressing or undressing

---

of dyspnea on a scale of 1 to 10, in which 1 means no dyspnea and 10 means the worst he has experienced. Then ask him to rate the level that day.

Next, ask the patient to grade his dyspnea as it relates to activity (see *Grading dyspnea*). In addition, you might also ask these questions:
• What do you do to relieve the dyspnea?
• How well does it work?

Ortho who?

A patient with orthopnea (shortness of breath when lying down) tends to sleep with his upper body elevated. Ask this patient how many pillows he uses. The answer describes the severity of orthopnea. For example, a patient who uses three pillows can be said to have "three-pillow orthopnea."

Cough it up

Ask the patient with a cough these questions: If the cough is a chronic problem, has it changed recently? If so, how? What makes the cough better? What makes it worse? Is the cough productive?

Make yourself productive

When a patient produces sputum, ask him to estimate the amount produced in teaspoons or some other common measurement. Also ask him these questions: At what time of day do you cough most often? What is the color and consistency of the sputum? If sputum is a chronic problem, has it changed recently? If so, how? Do you cough up blood? If so, how much and how often?

Whistle while you work

If a patient wheezes, ask these questions: When does wheezing occur? What makes you wheeze? Do you wheeze loudly enough for others to hear it? What helps stop your wheezing?

A pain in the chest

If the patient has chest pain, ask him these questions: Where is the pain? What does it feel like? Is it sharp, stabbing, burning, or aching? Does it move to another area? How long does it last? What causes it to occur? What makes it better?

Chest pain that occurs from a respiratory problem is usually the result of pleural inflammation, inflammation of the costochondral junctions, soreness of chest muscles because of coughing, or indigestion. Less common causes of pain include rib or vertebral fractures caused by coughing or by osteoporosis.

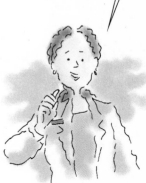

If the patient complains of chest pain, ask him to describe the pain, along with what causes the pain and what makes it better.

Dredging up the past

Remember to look at the patient's medical and family history, being particularly watchful for a smoking habit, allergies, previous operations, and respiratory diseases, such as pneumonia and tuberculosis.

Also, ask about environmental exposure to irritants such as asbestos. People who work in mining, construction, or chemical manufacturing are commonly exposed to environmental irritants. (See *Listen and learn*, then *teach*, page 24.)

Listen and learn, *then* teach

Listening to what your patient says about his respiratory problems will help you know when he needs patient education. The following typical responses indicate that the patient needs to know more about self-care techniques.

"Whenever I feel breathless, I just take a shot of my inhaler."
  This patient needs to know more about proper use of an inhaler and when to call the doctor.

"If I feel all congested, I just smoke a cigarette, and then I can cough up that phlegm!"
  This patient needs to know about the dangers of cigarette smoking.

"None of the other guys wear a mask when we're working."
  This patient needs to know the importance of wearing an appropriate safety mask when working around heavy dust and particles in the air, such as sawdust or powders.

Performing the physical examination

Any patient can develop a respiratory disorder. By using systematic assessment, you can detect subtle or obvious respiratory changes. The depth of your assessment depends on several factors, including the patient's primary health problem and his risk of developing respiratory complications.

A physical examination of the respiratory system follows four steps: inspection, palpation, percussion, and auscultation. Before you begin, make sure the room is well lit and warm.

First impressions

Make a few observations about the patient as soon as you enter the room. Note how the patient is seated, which is likely to be the position most comfortable for him. Take note of his level of awareness and general appearance. Does he appear relaxed? Anxious? Uncomfortable? Is he

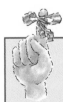

Memory jogger

To remember the order in which you should perform assessment of the respiratory system, just think, "I'll Properly Perform Assessment."

Inspection
Palpation
Percussion
Auscultation

having trouble breathing? Be sure to include these observations in your final assessment.

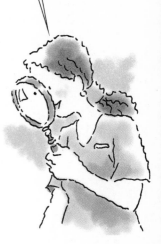

I love honing my inspection skills during a respiratory assessment.

Inspecting the chest

Before you further assess the patient, be sure to introduce yourself and explain why you're there. Then help the patient into an upright position. The patient should be undressed from the waist up or clothed in an examination gown that allows you access to his chest.

Taking a backward view

Examine the back of the chest first, using inspection, palpation, percussion, and auscultation. Always compare one side with the other. Then examine the front of the chest using the same sequence. The patient can lie back when you examine the front of the chest if that's more comfortable for him.

Beauty in symmetry

Note masses or scars that indicate trauma or surgery. Look for chest wall symmetry. Both sides of the chest should be equal at rest and expand equally as the patient inhales. The diameter of the chest, from front to back, should be about half the width of the chest. (See *Identifying chest deformities*, page 26.)

A new angle

Also, look at the angle between the ribs and the sternum at the point immediately above the xiphoid process. This angle — the costal angle — should be less than 90 degrees in an adult. The angle will be larger if the chest wall is chronically expanded because of an enlargement of the intercostal muscles, as can happen with chronic obstructive pulmonary disease.

Breathing easy

To find the patient's respiratory rate, count for a full minute — longer if you note abnormalities. Don't tell him what you're doing or he might alter his natural breathing pattern.

Adults normally breathe at a rate of 12 to 20 breaths/minute. An infant's breathing rate may reach up to 40 breaths/minute. The respiratory pattern should be even,

Identifying chest deformities

As you inspect the patient's chest, note deviations in size and shape. The illustrations below show a normal adult chest and four common chest deformities.

| **Normal adult chest** | **Barrel chest** Increased anteroposterior diameter | **Pigeon chest** Anteriorly displaced sternum | **Funnel chest** Depressed lower sternum | **Thoracic kyphoscoliosis** Raised shoulder and scapula, thoracic convexity, and flared interspaces |

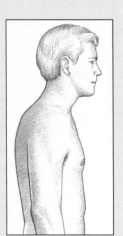 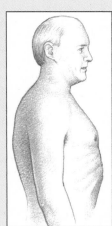 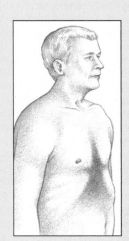 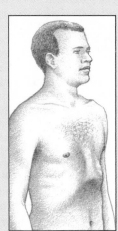 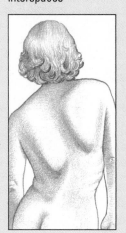

coordinated, and regular, with occasional sighs. (See *Spotting abnormal respiratory patterns.*)

An uneven exchange

Watch for paradoxical, or uneven, movement of the chest wall. Paradoxical movement may appear as an abnormal collapse of part of the chest wall when the patient inhales or an abnormal expansion when the patient exhales. In either case, this uneven movement indicates a loss of normal chest wall function.

Muscles in motion

When the patient inhales, his diaphragm should descend and the intercostal muscles should contract. This dual motion causes the abdomen to push out and the lower ribs to expand laterally.

Spotting abnormal respiratory patterns

Here are typical characteristics of the most common abnormal respiratory patterns.

Tachypnea
Shallow breathing with increased respiratory rate

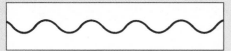

Bradypnea
Decreased rate but regular breathing

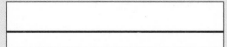

Apnea
Absence of breathing; may be periodic

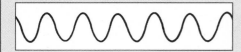

Hyperpnea
Deep breathing at a normal rate

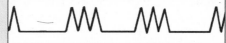

Kussmaul's respirations
Rapid, deep breathing without pauses; in adults, more than 20 breaths/minute; breathing usually sounds labored with deep breaths that resemble sighs

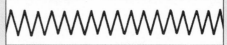

Cheyne-Stokes respirations
Breaths that gradually become faster and deeper than normal, then slower, during a 30- to 170-second period; alternates with 20- to 60-second periods of apnea

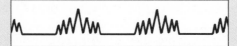

Biot's respirations
Rapid, deep breathing with abrupt pauses between each breath; equal depth to each breath

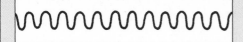

When the patient exhales, his abdomen and ribs return to their resting position. The upper chest shouldn't move much. Accessory muscles may hypertrophy, indicating frequent use. Frequent use of accessory muscles may be normal in some athletes; for other patients, however, it indicates a respiratory problem, particularly when the patient purses his lips and flares his nostrils when breathing.

Inspecting related structures

Inspection of the skin, tongue, mouth, fingers, and nail beds may also provide information about respiratory status.

An unbecoming color

Skin color varies considerably among patients, but in all cases a patient with a bluish tint to his skin and mucous membranes is considered cyanotic. Cyanosis, which occurs when oxygenation to the tissues is poor, is a late sign of hypoxemia.

The most reliable place to check for cyanosis is the tongue and mucous membranes of the mouth. A chilled patient may have cyanotic nail beds, nose, or ears, indicating low blood flow to those areas but not necessarily to major organs.

Clubbing clues

When you check the fingers, look for clubbing, a possible sign of long-term hypoxia. A fingernail normally enters the skin at an angle of less than 180 degrees. When clubbing occurs, the angle is greater than or equal to 180 degrees.

Palpating the chest

Palpation of the chest provides some important information about the respiratory system and the processes involved in breathing. (See *Performing chest palpation*.)

Here's what to look for when palpating the chest.

Snap, crackle, pop

The chest wall should feel smooth, warm, and dry. Crepitus indicates subcutaneous air in the chest, an abnormal condition. Crepitus feels like puffed-rice cereal crackling under the skin and indicates that air is leaking from the airways or lungs.

If a patient has a chest tube, you may find a small amount of subcutaneous air around the insertion site. If the patient has no chest tube or the area of crepitus is getting larger, alert the doctor immediately.

Tender touch

Gentle palpation shouldn't cause the patient pain. If the patient complains of chest pain, try to find a painful area

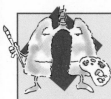

Inspired work

Performing chest palpation

To palpate the chest, place the palm of your hand (or hands) lightly over the thorax, as shown below left. Palpate for tenderness, alignment, bulging, and retractions of the chest and intercostal spaces. Assess the patient for crepitus, especially around drainage sites. Repeat this procedure on the patient's back.

Next, use the pads of your fingers, as shown below right, to palpate the front and back of the thorax. Pass your fingers over the ribs and any scars, lumps, lesions, or ulcerations. Note the skin temperature, turgor, and moisture. Also note tenderness and bony or subcutaneous crepitus. The muscles should feel firm and smooth.

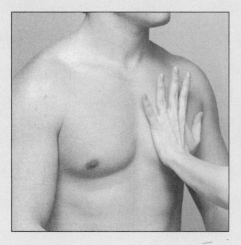

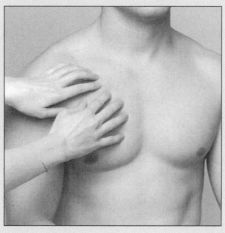

on the chest wall. Painful costochondral joints are typically located at the midclavicular line or next to the sternum. Rib or vertebral fractures are quite painful over the fracture, though pain may radiate around the chest as well. Pain may also be caused by sore muscles as a result of protracted coughing. A collapsed lung may also cause pain.

Strange vibrations

Palpate for tactile fremitus, palpable vibrations caused by the transmission of air through the bronchopulmonary system. Fremitus is decreased over areas where pleural fluid collects, at times when the patient speaks softly, and within pneumothorax, atelectasis, and emphysema. Frem-

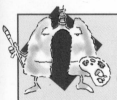

Inspired work

Checking for tactile fremitus

When you check the back of the thorax for tactile fremitus, ask the patient to fold his arms across his chest. This movement shifts the scapulae out of the way.

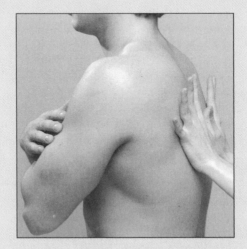

What to do

Check for tactile fremitus by lightly placing your open palms on both sides of the patient's back, as shown at right, without touching his back with his fingers. Ask the patient to repeat the phrase "ninety-nine" loud enough to produce palpable vibrations. Then palpate the front of the chest using the same hand positions.

What the results mean

Vibrations that feel more intense on one side than the other indicate tissue consolidation on that side. Less intense vibrations may indicate emphysema, pneumothorax, or pleural effu- sion. Faint or no vibrations in the upper posterior thorax may indicate bronchial obstruction or a fluid-filled pleural space.

itus is increased normally over the large bronchial tubes and abnormally over areas in which alveoli are filled with fluid or exudate, as happens in pneumonia. (See *Checking for tactile fremitus*.)

Expanding your horizons

To evaluate the patient's chest wall symmetry and expansion, place your hands on the front of the chest wall with your thumbs touching each other at the second intercostal space. As the patient inhales deeply, watch your thumbs. They should separate simultaneously and equally to a distance several centimeters away from the sternum.

Repeat the measurement at the fifth intercostal space. The same measurement may be made on the back of the chest near the tenth rib.

Warning signs

The patient's chest may expand asymmetrically if he has pleural effusion, atelectasis, pneumonia, or pneumothorax. Chest expansion may be decreased at the level of the diaphragm if the patient has emphysema, respiratory depression, diaphragm paralysis, atelectasis, obesity, or ascites.

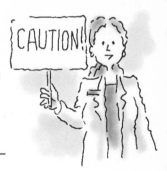

Percussing the chest

You'll percuss the chest to find the boundaries of the lungs, to determine whether the lungs are filled with air or fluid or solid material, and to evaluate the distance the diaphragm travels between the patient's inhalation and exhalation. (See *Performing chest percussion.*)

Percussion instruments

Percussion allows you to assess structures as deep as 3″ (7.6 cm). You'll hear different percussion sounds in different areas of the chest. (See *Percussion sounds*, page 32.)

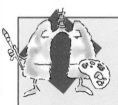

Inspired work

Performing chest percussion

To percuss the chest, hyperextend the middle finger of your left hand if you're right-handed or the middle finger of your right hand if you're left-handed. Place your hand firmly on the patient's chest. Use the tip of the middle finger of your dominant hand—your right hand if you're right-handed, left hand if you're left-handed—to tap on the middle finger of your other hand just below the distal joint (as shown at right).

The movement should come from the wrist of your dominant hand, not your elbow or upper arm. Keep the fingernail you use for tapping short so you won't hurt yourself. Follow the standard percussion sequence over the front and back chest walls.

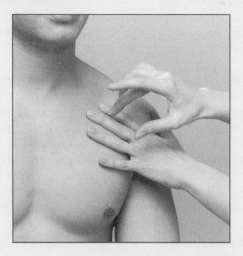

Percussion sounds

Use this chart to become more comfortable with percussion and to help interpret percussion sounds quickly. Learn the different percussion sounds by practicing on yourself, your patients, and any other person willing to help.

Sound	Description	Clinical significance
Flat	Short, soft, high-pitched, extremely dull, found over the thigh	Consolidation, as in atelectasis and extensive pleural effusion
Dull	Medium in intensity and pitch, moderate length, thudlike, found over the liver	Solid area, as in pleural effusion
Resonant	Long, loud, low-pitched, hollow	Normal lung tissue
Hyperresonant	Very loud, lower-pitched, found over the stomach	Hyperinflated lung, as in emphysema or pneumothorax
Tympanic	Loud, high-pitched, moderate length, musical, drumlike, found over a puffed-out cheek	Air collection, as in a gastric air bubble or air in the intestines

Percussing the chest is like making music with a drum. Different areas of the chest produce different sounds.

You may also hear different sounds after certain treatments. For example, if your patient has atelectasis and you percuss his chest before chest physiotherapy, you'll hear a high-pitched, dull, soft sound. After physiotherapy, you should hear a low-pitched, hollow sound. In all cases, make sure you use other assessment techniques to confirm percussion findings. (See *Double-check percussion findings.*)

Ringing with resonance

You'll hear resonant sounds over normal lung tissue, which you should find over most of the chest. In the left front chest from the third or fourth intercostal space at the sternum to the third or fourth intercostal space at the midclavicular line, you should hear a dull sound. Percussion is dull there because that's the space occupied by the heart. Resonance resumes at the sixth intercostal space. The sequence of sounds in the back is slightly different. (See *Percussion sequences.*)

A sour note

When you hear hyperresonance during percussion, it means that you've found an area of increased air in the lung or pleural space. Expect hyperresonance with pneumothorax, acute asthma, bullous emphysema (large holes in the lungs from alveolar destruction), or gastric distention that pushes up on the diaphragm.

When you hear abnormal dullness, it means that you've found areas of decreased air in the lungs. Expect abnormal dullness in the presence of pleural fluid, consolidation, atelectasis, or a tumor.

Sinking to a new level

Percussion also allows you to assess how much the diaphragm moves during inspiration and expiration. The normal diaphragm descends 1¼″ to 2″ (3 to 5 cm) when the patient inhales. The diaphragm doesn't move as far in

Double-check percussion findings

Use other assessment findings to verify the results of respiratory percussion. For example, if an X-ray report on a patient with chronic obstructive pulmonary disease indicates findings consistent with emphysema, you should hear low-pitched, loud booming sounds when you percuss the chest.

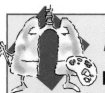

Inspired work

Percussion sequences

Follow these percussion sequences to distinguish between normal and abnormal sounds in the patient's lungs. Remember to compare sound variations from one side with the other as you proceed. Carefully describe abnormal sounds you hear and include their locations. You'll follow the same sequences for auscultation.

Anterior

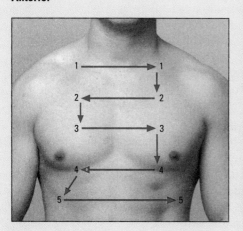

Posterior

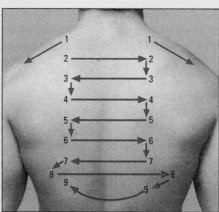

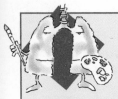

Inspired work

Measuring diaphragm movement

You can measure how much the diaphragm moves by asking the patient to exhale. Percuss the back on one side to locate the upper edge of the diaphragm, the point at which normal lung resonance changes to dullness. Use a pen to mark the spot indicating the position of the diaphragm at full expiration on that side of the back.

Then ask the patient to inhale as deeply as possible. Percuss the back when the patient has breathed in fully until you locate the diaphragm. Use the pen to mark this spot as well. Repeat on the opposite side of the back.

Measure

Use a ruler or tape measure to determine the distance between the marks. The distance, normally 1¼″ to 2″ (3 to 5 cm) long, should be equal on both the right and left sides.

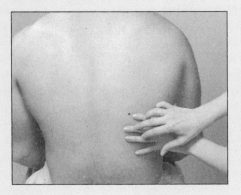

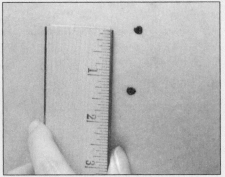

patients with emphysema, respiratory depression, diaphragm paralysis, atelectasis, obesity, or ascites. (See *Measuring diaphragm movement*.)

Auscultating the chest

As air moves through the bronchi, it creates sound waves that travel to the chest wall. The sounds produced by breathing change as air moves from larger airways to smaller airways. Sounds also change if they pass through fluid, mucus, or narrowed airways. Auscultation helps you to determine the condition of the alveoli and surrounding pleura.

To gain the most information possible, make sure you perform your assessment in a quiet environment. Also, keep in mind that following a proper sequence and comparing sounds can enhance your assessment findings.

Quiet on the set!

Breath sounds have a wide range of sound frequencies, many near the lower threshold of human hearing. Consequently, the environment for auscultation should be as quiet as possible so that you can hear breath sounds clearly and distinctly. Close the door to the room and eliminate extraneous noises and conversations; turn off televisions and radios. You'll need to develop good concentration skills so that noises from such devices as I.V. pumps, oxygen delivery systems, and ventilators don't interfere with auscultation. (See *Using a stethoscope*, page 36.)

Fine-tuning your reception

During auscultation, press the diaphragm of the stethoscope firmly against the patient's chest wall over the intercostal spaces. Try not to listen directly over bone. Never listen through clothing, which impedes or alters sound transmission. Avoid other extraneous sounds such as those caused by the stethoscope rubbing against bed rails or other objects. (See *Minimizing outside noise*, page 36.)

A one, and a two...

The auscultatory sequence for the posterior chest wall surface includes 10 different sites. (See *Auscultatory sequence*, page 37.) The first site is above the left scapula over the lung apex. From there, the auscultatory sequence follows a pattern that progresses downward from the lung apices to the bases. This pattern covers the entire posterior chest wall surface and includes a comparison of sounds heard over the same auscultatory site over both the right and left lungs. Sites 5, 7, and 10 are located over the lateral chest wall surfaces.

The anterior chest wall auscultatory sequence includes nine sites and follows the same pattern as the posterior chest wall sequence. The pattern also includes sites over the lateral chest wall surfaces.

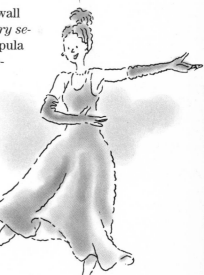

Following an auscultatory sequence is similar to dancing a waltz...ONE, two, three; ONE, two three...

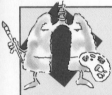

Inspired work

Using a stethoscope

Proper stethoscope use is an important part of your respiratory assessment. The stethoscope allows you to hear breath sounds transmitted through the chest wall. Most stethoscopes have a diaphragm and a bell, with one or two tubes leading to the binaural headpiece and earpieces. The diaphragm is used to listen for high-pitched breath sounds; the bell is used to listen for low-pitched breath sounds. Applying the stethoscope firmly to the chest wall amplifies high-frequency sounds. However, if too much pressure is applied when using the bell, the stretched skin functions as a diaphragm and filters out low-pitched sounds.

Checking the equipment
The stethoscope tubing should be no longer than 10″ to 12″ (25 to 30 cm). It should be tightly attached to the binaural headpiece and the stethoscope body to prevent air leakage, which could result in the loss of sound energy. The earpieces must be securely attached to the binaural headpiece, which removes extraneous noise from the environment, to avoid any sound loss. They should fit tightly and should be placed into the ears in an anterior direction so that they conform to the direction of the ear canals. Check the stethoscope to ensure that the diaphragm and bell are locked into place prior to auscultating. Some stethoscopes have a rotating bell or diaphragm that may become disengaged; this can block or muffle breath sounds.

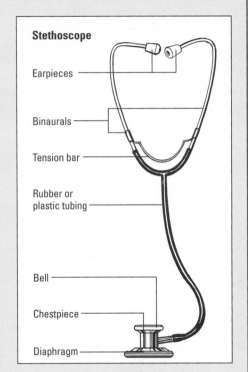

Stethoscope

Earpieces

Binaurals

Tension bar

Rubber or plastic tubing

Bell

Chestpiece

Diaphragm

Take a deep breath

If the patient is alert and healthy, begin auscultation with the patient sitting upright and leaning slightly forward. Position yourself behind the patient. Ask the patient to breathe through an open mouth, slightly deeper than usual, through several respiratory cycles. (*Note:* If the patient is extremely dyspneic, don't ask him to take deeper breaths. In this case, begin auscultating for breath sounds at the bilateral lung bases.)

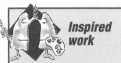

Inspired work

Minimizing outside noise

If the patient has a very hairy chest or back, lightly dampen the chest hair and hold the stethoscope firmly against the skin to minimize the crackling noises produced by dry hair.

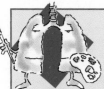

Inspired work

Auscultatory sequence

Follow these auscultation sequences to distinguish between normal and abnormal sounds in the patient's lungs. Remember to compare sound variations from one side with the other as you proceed. Carefully describe abnormal sounds you hear and include locations.

Posterior auscultatory sequence

Anterior auscultatory sequence

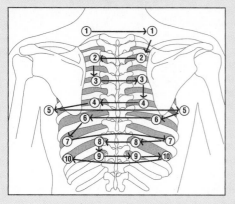
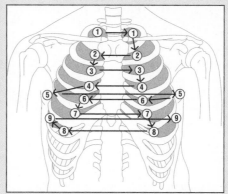

Slow but steady

Place the diaphragm of the stethoscope over the left lung apex, and listen for at least one complete respiratory cycle. Then move the diaphragm to the same site over the right lung. Compare the breath sounds heard over these same locations. Continue in this manner, making contralateral comparisons at each auscultatory site.

After you have auscultated the entire posterior chest wall and parts of the lateral chest walls, move to the front of the patient. Have the patient place his arms at his sides and breathe through an open mouth, slightly deeper than usual, as you listen to breath sounds over the anterior chest wall. You can obtain additional information about tracheal sounds by auscultating over the sternum, larynx, and mouth. (See *The better to hear you*.)

Is this normal?

During auscultation, you'll hear four types of breath sounds over normal lungs. The type of sound you hear

---

The better to hear you

You may roll comatose, critically ill, or bedridden patients from one side to the other to auscultate dependent lung regions. Listen initially over dependent lung regions because gravity-dependent secretions or fluids may produce abnormal sounds that sometimes disappear when the patient is turned, breathes deeply, or coughs.

Locations of normal breath sounds

These photographs show the normal locations of different types of breath sounds.

Anterior thorax

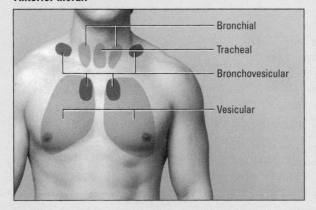

- Bronchial
- Tracheal
- Bronchovesicular
- Vesicular

Posterior thorax

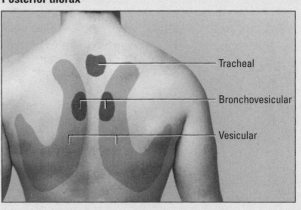

- Tracheal
- Bronchovesicular
- Vesicular

depends on where you listen (see *Locations of normal breath sounds*):

- Tracheal breath sounds, heard over the trachea, are harsh and discontinuous. They occur when a patient inhales or exhales.
- Bronchial breath sounds, usually heard next to the trachea, are loud, high-pitched, and discontinuous. They're loudest when the patient exhales.
- Bronchovesicular sounds, heard when the patient inhales or exhales, are medium-pitched and continuous. They're best heard over the upper third of the sternum and between the scapulae.
- Vesicular sounds, heard over the rest of the lungs, are soft and low-pitched. They're prolonged during inhalation and shortened during exhalation.

(See *Characteristics of breath sounds*.)

I can't hear you!

If you hear diminished but normal breath sounds in both lungs, the patient may have emphysema, atelectasis, severe broncho-spasm, or shallow breathing. If you hear breath sounds in one lung only, the patient may have pleural effusion, pneumothorax, a tumor, or mucus plugs in the airways. In such cases, the doctor may order pulmonary function tests to further assess the patient's con-

Characteristics of breath sounds

Use this chart to help you recognize patterns of breath sounds by their intensity, pitch, and duration of inspiratory and expiratory phases. Note that the thickness of the bars indicates intensity; the steeper an incline, the higher the pitch.

Breath sound	Duration of sounds	Intensity of expiratory sound	Pitch of expiratory sound	Location where normally heard
Vesicular	Inspiratory sounds last longer than expiratory ones.	Soft	Relatively low	Over most of the lungs
Bronchovesicular	Inspiratory and expiratory sounds are about equal.	Intermediate	Intermediate	Commonly in the first and second interspaces anteriorly and between the scapulae
Bronchial	Expiratory sounds last longer than inspiratory ones.	Loud	Relatively high	Over the manubrium, if heard at all
Tracheal	Inspiratory and expiratory sounds are about equal.	Very loud	Relatively high	Over the trachea in the neck

dition. (See *Interpreting pulmonary function test results*, page 40.)

Sounding board

Classify each sound according to its intensity, location, pitch, duration, and characteristic. Note whether the sound occurs when the patient inhales, exhales, or both. If you hear a sound in an area other than that in which you would expect to hear it, consider the sound abnormal.

For example, bronchial or bronchovesicular breath sounds found in an area where vesicular breath sounds would normally be heard indicates that the alveoli and small bronchioles in that area might be filled with fluid or exudate, as occurs in pneumonia and atelectasis. You won't hear vesicular sounds in those areas because no air is moving through the small airways.

Voicing your complaints

Finally, check for vocal fremitus, which is the sound produced by chest vibrations as the patient speaks. Abnormal

Interpreting pulmonary function test results

You may need to interpret results of pulmonary function tests in your assessment of a patient's respiratory status. Use the chart below as a guide to common pulmonary function tests.

Restrictive and obstructive

The chart mentions restrictive and obstructive defects. A restrictive defect is one in which a person can't inhale a normal amount of air. It may occur with chest wall deformities, neuromuscular diseases, or acute respiratory tract infections.

An obstructive defect is one in which something obstructs the flow of air into or out of the lungs. It may occur with a disease such as asthma, chronic bronchitis, emphysema, or cystic fibrosis.

Test	Implications
Tidal volume (V_T) Amount of air inhaled or exhaled during normal breathing	Decreased V_T may indicate restrictive disease and requires further tests, such as full pulmonary function studies or chest X-rays.
Minute volume (MV) Amount of air breathed per minute	Normal MV can occur in emphysema. Decreased MV may indicate other diseases such as pulmonary edema.
Inspiratory reserve volume (IRV) Amount of air inhaled after normal inspiration	Abnormal IRV alone doesn't indicate respiratory dysfunction. IRV decreases during normal exercise.
Expiratory reserve volume (ERV) Amount of air that can be exhaled after normal expiration	ERV varies, even in healthy people.
Vital capacity (VC) Amount of air that can be exhaled after maximum inspiration	Normal or increased VC with decreased flow rates may indicate reduction in functional pulmonary tissue. Decreased VC with normal or increased flow rates may indicate decreased respiratory effort, decreased thoracic expansion, or limited movement of the diaphragm.
Inspiratory capacity (IC) Amount of air that can be inhaled after normal expiration	Decreased IC indicates restrictive disease.
Forced vital capacity (FVC) Amount of air that can be exhaled after maximum inspiration	Decreased FVC indicates flow resistance in the respiratory system from obstructive disease, such as chronic bronchitis, emphysema, and asthma.
Forced expiratory volume (FEV) Volume of air exhaled in the first (FEV_1), second (FEV_2), or third (FEV_3) FVC maneuver	Decreased FEV_1 and increased FEV_2 and FEV_3 may indicate obstructive disease. Decreased or normal FEV_1 may indicate restrictive disease.

transmission of voice sounds—the most common of which are bronchophony, egophony, and whispered pectoriloquy—may occur over consolidated areas. (See *Normal and altered breath and voice sounds.*)

To check for bronchophony, ask the patient to say "ninety-nine" or "blue moon." Over normal lung tissue, the words sound muffled. Over consolidated areas, the words sound unusually loud. Next, to check for egophony, ask the patient to say "E." Over normal lung tissue, the sound

Normal and altered breath and voice sounds

The findings in a normally air-filled lung and an airless lung are summarized below.

	Normally air-filled lung	**Airless lung, as in lobar pneumonia**
Breath sounds	Predominantly vesicular	Bronchial or bronchovesicular over the involved area
Transmitted voice sounds	Spoken words muffled and indistinct	Spoken words louder, clearer (bronchophony)
	Spoken "ee" heard as "ee"	Spoken "ee" heard as "ay" (egophony)
	Whispered words faint and indistinct, if heard at all	Whispered words louder, clearer (whispered pectoriloquy)
Tactile fremitus	Normal	Increased

is muffled. Over consolidated lung tissue, it will sound like the letter *a.* Then ask the patient to whisper "1, 2, 3." Over normal lung tissue, the numbers will be almost indistinguishable. Over consolidated lung tissue, the numbers will be loud and clear.

Final exams

A patient with abnormal findings during a respiratory assessment may be further evaluated using such diagnostic tests as arterial blood gas analysis and pulmonary function tests.

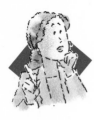

Quick quiz

1.   Paradoxical chest wall movement:
    A.   is normal.
    B.   indicates a loss of chest wall function.
    C.   is noted only when the patient exhales.
    D.   appears even.

Answer: B. Paradoxical or uneven chest wall movement indicates a loss of chest wall function. It may appear as an abnormal collapse of part of the chest wall when the patient inhales or an abnormal expansion when the patient exhales.

2.   Crepitus indicates:
    A.   air leakage from the airways or lungs.
    B.   the presence of subcutaneous air in the chest, which is normal.
    C.   a malfunctioning chest tube.
    D.   fluid in the pleural space.

Answer: A. Crepitus indicates that air is leaking from the airways or lungs. Subcutaneous air in the chest is abnormal. However, if the patient has a chest tube, you may find a small amount of subcutaneous air around the insertion site. If the patient has no chest tube, alert the doctor immediately.

3. Harsh, discontinuous breath sounds are normally heard:
- A. in the lower lobes.
- B. over the upper third of the sternum and between the scapulae.
- C. at the bases of the lungs.
- D. over the trachea.

Answer: D. Harsh, discontinuous breath sounds are normally heard over the trachea. They occur when a patient inhales or exhales.

4. High-pitched breath sounds are best heard by using:
- A. the diaphragm of the stethoscope.
- B. the bell of the stethoscope.
- C. both the bell and the diaphragm of the stethoscope.
- D. a stethoscope with tubing at least 20″ (51 cm) in length.

Answer: A. The diaphragm is used to listen for high-pitched breath sounds; the bell is used to listen for low-pitched breath sounds. Applying the stethoscope firmly to the chest wall amplifies high-frequency sounds. However, if too much pressure is applied when using the bell, the stretched skin functions as a diaphragm and filters out low-pitched sounds. Tubing length isn't a factor in hearing high-pitched sounds, but it shouldn't be longer than 10″ to 12″ (25 to 30 cm).

5. To auscultate the breath sounds of a patient who's alert and healthy:
- A. have the patient lie on his side and then roll him from one side to the other as you listen.
- B. have the patient sit upright and lean slightly forward; stand behind the patient to auscultate the posterior first.
- C. have the patient first lie on his back and then roll onto his abdomen.
- D. you may listen through clothing as long as the patient sits upright and leans slightly forward.

Answer: B. The alert, healthy patient should sit upright and lean slightly forward. Position yourself behind the patient. After auscultating the entire posterior chest wall and parts of the lateral chest walls, move to the front of the patient. Never listen through clothing, which impedes or alters sound transmission.

Scoring

☆☆☆ If you answered all five questions correctly, excellent!
        You've left us breathless with your expertise.

☆☆ If you answered four questions correctly, hooray! You're
        our resident respiratory guru.

☆ If you answered fewer than four questions correctly, no
        problem! Just do another assessment of this chapter.

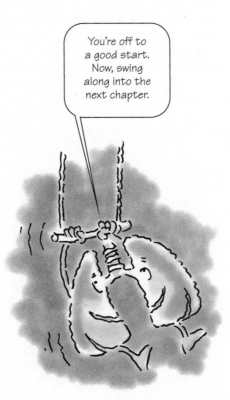

You're off to a good start. Now, swing along into the next chapter.

Introduction to breath sounds

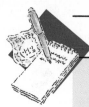

Just the facts

In this chapter, you'll learn:

♦ the origin of breath sounds

♦ the concepts of airway dynamics and airflow patterns

♦ factors affecting breath sounds

♦ classifications for normal, voice, and adventitious sounds.

Breath sounds at a glance

Breath sounds result as air moves through the airways of the respiratory tract. The diameter of the airway, pressure changes in the airway, and vibrations of solid tissue all affect the sound produced. This chapter discusses the properties that affect airflow and sound transmission as well as the normal and abnormal breath sounds that result. Documenting your findings and structuring an effective care plan are also reviewed.

Understanding airflow

The way air flows through the respiratory system influences the types of sounds heard during auscultation. Understanding airway dynamics and airflow patterns are a key first step in understanding breath sounds.

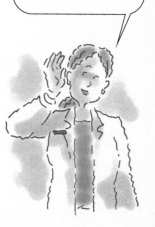

Note that the diameter of the airway, pressure changes in the airway, and vibrations of solid tissue all affect the sound produced as air moves through the respiratory tract.

Airway dynamics

When the chest begins to expand during inspiration, the pressure within the pleural space (intrapleural pressure) decreases. The lungs stretch until the pressure within the alveoli (intrapulmonary pressure) drops below atmospheric pressure. This change in pressure draws air into the lungs. At the same time, the airways widen, decreasing resistance to the incoming air.

Feeling the pressure

During expiration, the lungs, which were stretched during inspiration, contract. The pressure within the pleural space and the lungs increases until it rises above atmospheric pressure, driving air out of the lungs. As air leaves the lungs, the pressures fall once again. (See *A close look at breathing*.)

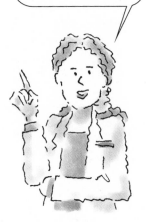

Keep in mind that the lungs and chest don't expand because of the entry of air. Rather, it's the difference in pressures between the atmosphere and the lungs that drives air into the lungs.

Airflow patterns

The respiratory tract consists of an intricate network of branching airways of various diameters, some of which have irregular wall surfaces. These factors affect the pattern of airflow and the resultant breath sounds. Airflow may be turbulent, circular (called *vortices*), or laminar. (See *Comparing airflow patterns*, page 48.)

Turbulent airflow

During rapid airflow movement, air molecules circulate randomly and collide against airway walls and each other, producing an eddying pattern. The colliding air molecules produce rapid pressure changes within the airway, which produces sound. This type of airflow—called *turbulent airflow*—occurs in the trachea, mainstem bronchi, and other larger airways.

Circular airflow

As air flows into the lungs, it must abruptly change direction in the branching airways. As it does so, it separates into layers, each moving at a different speed. The shearing force of the high-speed airstream against the slower airstream triggers a circular airflow, or vortices. This air-

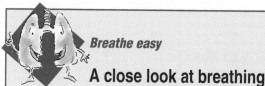

Breathe easy

A close look at breathing

These illustrations show how mechanical forces, such as movement of the diaphragm and intercostal muscles, produce a breath. A plus sign (+) indicates positive pressure, and a minus sign (–) indicates negative pressure.

At rest
- Inspiratory muscles relax.
- Atmospheric pressure is maintained in the tracheobronchial tree.
- No air movement occurs.

Inhalation
- Inspiratory muscles contract.
- The diaphragm descends.
- Negative alveolar pressure is maintained.
- Air moves into the lungs.

Exhalation
- Inspiratory muscles relax, causing the lungs to recoil to their resting size and position.
- The diaphragm ascends.
- Positive alveolar pressure is maintained.
- Air moves out of the lungs.

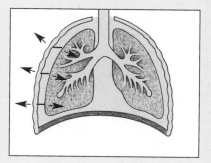
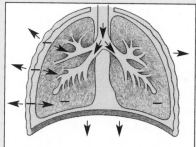
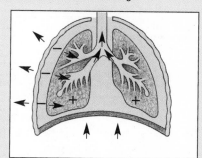

flow pattern generates sound as the flow of air carries the vortices downstream.

Laminar airflow

In the small airways and respiratory bronchioles, airflow is slow and linear. This is called *laminar airflow*. No abrupt changes in pressure or airway wall movements occur to generate sound. Consequently, air movement in these areas produces no sound.

Comparing airflow patterns

The following illustrations show the three primary airflow patterns affecting airway dynamics.

Turbulent airflow

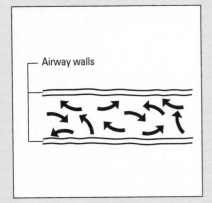

Circular airflow (vortices)

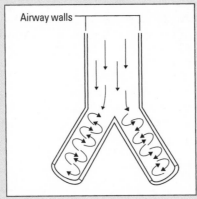

Laminar airflow

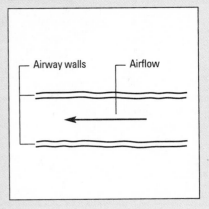

Understanding sound

Mechanical vibrations, sound damping, and impedance matching also affect the sounds heard during auscultation.

Mechanical vibrations

The mechanical vibrations of solid tissue also produce breath sounds. The speed at which these vibrations travel depends on whether they're traveling through air, fluid, or tissue. The frequency, intensity, and duration of these sounds can be measured.

Frequency

Frequency — measured in hertz — refers to the number of vibrations occurring per unit of time. Different frequencies produce the different sounds heard during auscultation. In clinical settings, the term *pitch* is used to describe sound frequency. High-pitched sounds have higher frequencies; low-pitched sounds have lower frequencies.

Intensity

Intensity refers to the loudness or softness of the vibrations that produce breath sounds. Intensity can be measured electronically by recording amplitude. Several factors affect intensity, including the type of structure that's vibrating as well as the distance and type of substance through which the vibrations must travel.

Duration

The duration of the vibrations that produce breath sounds can be measured in milliseconds. However, during auscultation, you'll note sounds as being long or short and as continuous or discontinuous.

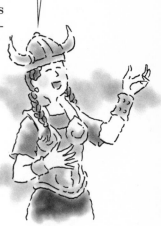

Remember, pitch refers to the frequency of a sound; intensity refers to the loudness or softness. When I sing, I'm loud and I have perfect pitch. La, la, la, la!

Sound damping

Depending on where you listen to breath sounds, certain sounds may be amplified while others are damped. For example, breath sounds arising from the same location in the lung have a higher pitch when heard at the mouth or over the trachea than when heard over the chest wall. This change in pitch occurs because high-pitched breath sounds are absorbed (damped) as they travel through the lungs and thorax.

Voice sounds are also affected by damping. The resonant qualities of the mouth, nasopharynx, paranasal sinuses, and chest cavity contribute to the pitch and intensity of voice sounds.

Impedance matching

Breath and voice sounds are normally filtered, or damped, when they travel through air, fluid, and tissue. How much the sound is damped depends on how much the substance resists sound transmission. This is known as *impedance*. When two substances with similar acoustical properties are next to each other, sound is transmitted effectively.

The match game

For example, consolidated areas enhance the transmission of breath sounds to the chest wall. This happens because the consolidating substance, such as an inflammatory exudate, collects in alveoli, replacing air with dense tis-

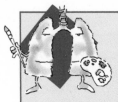

Inspired work

Auscultating an obese patient's lungs

In an obese person, a thickened chest wall increases the distance between the lung tissue and chest wall surface. For better results when auscultating an obese patient's lungs, ask him to take deep breaths through his open mouth while sitting upright or standing.

sue. The fluid-filled, airless lung tissue and the chest wall are acoustically well matched, and breath sounds travel more easily. On the other hand, if fluid (or solid tissue) collects between inflated lung segments, an impedance mismatch occurs. Therefore, breath and voice sounds are significantly filtered, reducing the sounds heard on auscultation.

Diseases that increase the impedance mismatch include pleural effusion and empyema. Obesity also causes diminished breath sounds because of the increased distance between the stethoscope and the lungs. (See *Auscultating an obese patient's lungs*.)

Because solid tissue transmits sound better than air or fluid, breath sounds, as well as spoken words, are louder than normal over areas of consolidation. If pus, fluid, or air fills the pleural space, breath sounds are quieter than normal.

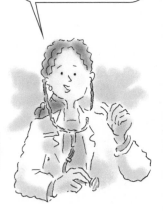

Classifying sounds

Both normal and abnormal breath sounds have certain recognizable characteristics. Airflow patterns, regional lung volume, distribution of ventilation, body position, and the site producing the sound all affect the sounds heard during auscultation. In many cases, you can link a normal breath sound to a specific site in the respiratory system. However, this isn't always possible.

Normal breath sounds

Normal breath sounds include tracheal, bronchial, vesicular, and bronchovesicular breath sounds.

Hitting the high notes

Tracheal and bronchial sounds, which result from turbulent airflow in the first divisions of the large airways, are loud and hollow (tubular) sounding. They're heard best over the trachea and mainstem bronchi throughout inspiration and expiration. **(1)** Tracheal breath sounds are described as harsh and high pitched. Bronchial breath sounds are described as loud and high pitched.

Feeling faint

Vesicular breath sounds are faint; they're best heard over other chest wall areas throughout inspiration and at the beginning of expiration. **(2)** These sounds may result from turbulent airflow in the first few divisions of the large airways. However, because these sounds change with different airflow rates and according to the distribution of ventilation in the lungs, the sounds may also originate in the peripheral airways. It's also possible for vesicular breath sounds to originate in the peripheral airways during inspiration and in the larger airways during expiration. (For more information, see chapter 4, Normal breath sounds.)

A happy medium

Bronchovesicular breath sounds are heard over areas between the mainstem bronchi and the smaller airways. They have a pitch and duration midway between tracheal and mainstem bronchial sounds. They're equally audible during inspiration and expiration.

Abnormal breath sounds

Disease processes that alter the airway or airflow dynamics produce abnormal breath sounds. The vibration of solid structures, airflow through narrowed airways, and abrupt changes in airway pressure may all produce abnormal breath sounds. Abnormal breath sounds include adventitious sounds as well as voice sounds.

Adventitious sounds

Adventitious sounds are a specific type of abnormal breath sound. There are two types of adventitious sounds: crackles and wheezes.

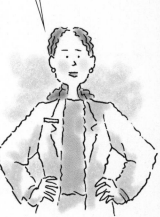

If a foreign body or secretions obstruct a bronchus, breath sounds distal to the obstruction will be diminished or absent.

Crackles and...

Coarse crackles (previously known as *rales* or *coarse rales*) are loud, low-pitched, explosive sounds that are discontinuous. **(39)** Fine crackles (previously known as *fine rales* or *crepitations*) also sound explosive and are discontinuous, but they have a shorter duration and a higher pitch and are less intense than coarse crackles. **(40)**

...wheezes and...

Wheezes (previously known as *sibilant rales* or *sibilant rhonchi*) are continuous and high-pitched, making a hissing or coughing-type sound. Wheezes commonly have a musical quality. **(41)** Low-pitched wheezes (previously known as *sonorous rales* or *sonorous rhonchi*) are continuous and low-pitched, making a snoring sound. **(42)**

...rhonchi, oh my!

You may still see the term *rhonchi* used to describe low-pitched wheezes. The term *rhonchi* describes a rough, rumbling, low-pitched sound, usually heard during expiration. At times, though, these sounds may be heard during inspiration. Rhonchi, which generally result when fluid or secretions partially block the large airways, may change or disappear when the patient coughs. (See *Comparing adventitious breath sounds.*)

Voice sounds

Voice sounds are vibrations produced by speech that are transmitted to the chest wall through the tracheobronchial tree. Abnormal transmission of voice sounds may occur over consolidated areas of lung tissue. Voice sounds are classified as bronchophony, egophony, and whispered pectoriloquy.

What did you say?

Voice sounds that have an increased tone or clarity in vocal resonance when auscultated over the chest wall are called *bronchophony*. In a healthy individual, bronchophony is similar to voice sounds heard through the neck. **(4)** Voice sounds that are spoken in a normal tone but are transmitted through the chest wall at a selectively amplified higher frequency are called *egophony*. **(5)** High-pitched whispered sounds transmitted through airless, consolidated lung tis-

Comparing adventitious breath sounds

The characteristics of discontinuous and continuous adventitious breath sounds are compared in the chart below. Note the timing of each sound during inspiration and expiration on the corresponding graphs.

Sound	Characteristics
Discontinuous sounds	
Fine crackles 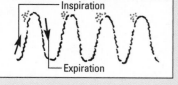	• Intermittent • Nonmusical • Soft • High-pitched • Short, cracking, popping sounds • Heard during inspiration (5 to 10 msec)
Coarse crackles 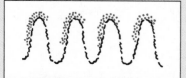	• Intermittent • Nonmusical • Loud • Low-pitched • Bubbling, gurgling sounds • Heard during early inspiration and possibly during expiration (20 to 30 msec)
Continuous sounds	
Wheezes 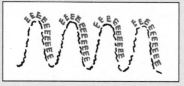	• Musical • High-pitched • Squeaking sounds • Predominantly heard during expiration but may also occur during inspiration
Rhonchi 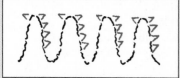	• Musical • Low-pitched • Snoring, moaning sounds • Heard during both inspiration and expiration, but are more prominent during expiration

sue are called *whispered pectoriloquy.* **(6)** (For more information, see chapter 6, Abnormal voice sounds.)

Documenting auscultation findings

Careful documentation of auscultation findings is essential for determining whether breath sounds have changed over time. After documentation, those findings are used to construct a nursing care plan.

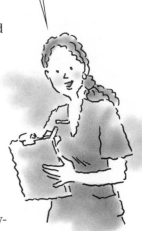

Document your auscultation findings carefully. That way, you'll be sure to pick up on any changes in the patient's breath sounds.

Proper documentation

Be sure to document the location, intensity, duration, and pitch of each auscultated breath in the patient's record. When documenting sound *location*, use anatomical landmarks, as well as lung bases and apices, as reference points. Note whether you heard the sound over the anterior, posterior, or lateral chest wall surface and whether you heard the sound over one (unilateral) or both (bilateral) lungs.

Terms of agreement

Describe sound *intensity* using such terms as "loud," "soft," "absent," "diminished," or "distant." Sound *duration* refers to the sound's timing within the respiratory cycle—that is, whether it's heard during inspiration, expiration, or both. Timing may be described as early, late, or throughout the respiratory cycle.

Record whether breath sounds have a high or a low *pitch.* This is especially important when documenting wheezes or crackles. In these instances, a difference in pitch helps differentiate between underlying disease processes.

Here's an example of how to document abnormal respiratory findings: "Late inspiratory fine crackles were heard over the right base posteriorly along the midscapular line, and coarse crackles were heard throughout inspiration and expiration over the left apex anteriorly near the midclavicular line."

Starting a care plan

Your initial assessment of breath sounds provides a baseline for ongoing respiratory assessment and care. After you document your initial auscultation findings, be ready to analyze the data and begin a care plan. As your patient's condition changes, so will the plan. Below you'll find some nursing diagnoses commonly used in patients with respiratory problems. For each diagnosis, you'll also find interventions and rationales. Remember to individualize each patient's care plan using an interdisciplinary approach.

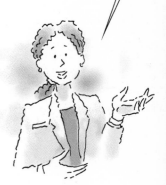

An up-to-date care plan ensures that the patient will receive the most appropriate care from each member of the health care team.

Ineffective breathing pattern related to decreased energy or increased fatigue

This diagnosis commonly applies to patients with such conditions as chronic obstructive pulmonary disease (COPD) and pulmonary embolus.

Expected outcomes
• Patient reports feeling comfortable when breathing.
• Patient achieves maximum lung expansion with adequate ventilation.
• Patient's respiratory rate remains within 5 breaths/minute of baseline.

Nursing interventions and rationales
• Auscultate breath sounds at least every 4 hours to detect decreased or adventitious breath sounds.
• Assess the adequacy of ventilation to detect early signs of respiratory compromise.
• Teach breathing techniques to help the patient improve ventilation.
• Teach relaxation techniques to help reduce the patient's anxiety and enhance his feeling of self-control.
• Administer bronchodilators to help relieve bronchospasm and wheezing.
• Administer oxygen as ordered to help relieve hypoxemia and respiratory distress.

Ineffective airway clearance related to tracheobronchial secretions or obstruction

This diagnosis commonly applies to patients with such conditions as asthma, COPD, interstitial lung disease, cystic fibrosis, and pneumonia.

Expected outcomes
- Patient coughs effectively.
- Patient's airway remains patent.
- Adventitious breath sounds are absent.

Nursing interventions and rationales
- Teach coughing techniques to promote chest expansion and ventilation, to enhance the clearance of secretions from airways, and to involve the patient in his own care.
- Perform postural drainage, percussion, and vibration to facilitate secretion movement.
- Encourage fluids to ensure adequate hydration and liquefy secretions.
- Give expectorants and mucolytics as ordered to enhance airway clearance.
- Provide an artificial airway as needed to maintain airway patency.

Impaired gas exchange related to altered oxygen supply or oxygen-carrying capacity of the blood

This diagnosis commonly applies to patients with acute respiratory failure, COPD, pneumonia, pulmonary embolism, and other respiratory problems.

Expected outcomes
- Patient's respiratory rate remains within 5 breaths/ minute of baseline.
- Patient has normal breath sounds.
- Patient's arterial blood gas (ABG) levels return to baseline.

Nursing interventions and rationales
- Give antibiotics, as ordered, and monitor their effectiveness in treating infection and improving alveolar expansion.

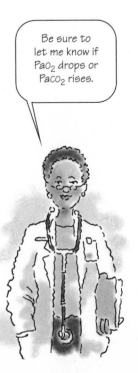

Be sure to let me know if Pao_2 drops or $Paco_2$ rises.

• Teach deep breathing and incentive spirometry to enhance lung expansion and ventilation.

• Monitor ABG values and notify the doctor immediately if the partial pressure of arterial oxygen (PaO_2) drops or the partial pressure of carbon dioxide ($PaCO_2$) rises. If needed, start mechanical ventilation to improve ventilation.

• Provide continuous positive airway pressure or positive end-expiratory pressure as needed to improve the driving pressure of oxygen across the alveolocapillary membrane, enhance arterial blood oxygenation, and increase lung compliance.

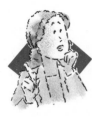

Quick quiz

1. When breath sounds travel through air-filled alveoli, fluid accumulations in the pleura, and solid structures such as bone, they're:

    A.   amplified.
    B.   eliminated.
    C.   distorted.
    D.   diminished.

Answer: D. Breath sounds are normally diminished and filtered as they travel through air-filled alveoli, fluid accumulations in the pleura, and solid structures such as bone.

2. Vortices are defined as:

    A.   normal breath sounds.
    B.   adventitious sounds.
    C.   airflow patterns.
    D.   equal pressure points.

Answer: C. Vortices are circular airflow patterns that generate sounds as the flow of air carries the vortices downstream.

3. High-pitched, whispered sounds transmitted through airless, consolidated space are called:

    A.   adventitious sounds.
    B.   egophony.
    C.   bronchophony.
    D.   whispered pectoriloquy.

Answer: D. High-pitched, whispered sounds transmitted through airless, consolidated space are called whispered pectoriloquy.

4. Which characteristics should be included when documenting breath sounds?
    A.   Location, intensity, duration, and pitch
    B.   Airflow pattern, pitch, and location
    C.   Duration, transmission, and intensity
    D.   Location, pitch, and source

Answer: A. Determine the location, intensity, duration, and pitch of each sound during auscultation and then document these characteristics in the patient's record.

5. Which continuous breath sound is high pitched and has a hissing or coughing sound?
    A.   Coarse crackles
    B.   Rhonchi
    C.   Wheezes
    D.   Fine crackles

Answer: C. Wheezes are continuous breath sounds that are high pitched and have a hissing or coughing sound.

Scoring

☆☆☆ If you answered all five questions correctly, outstanding! You've got the ins and outs of breathing down pat!

☆☆ If you answered four questions correctly, well done! It sounds like you have a healthy grasp on breath sounds!

☆ If you answered fewer than four questions correctly, don't develop respiratory distress. Why not flow through the chapter one more time?

4

Normal breath sounds

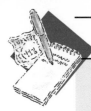

Just the facts

In this chapter, you'll learn:

♦ characteristics of normal breath sounds

♦ the origin of normal breath sounds

♦ conditions affecting normal breath sounds.

Normal breath sounds at a glance

Normal breath sounds result from airflow patterns in the respiratory system, associated pressure changes within the airways, and solid tissue vibrations. Various factors influence the sounds heard on auscultation. These include the distance between the source of the sound and the chest wall, the path of sound transmission, and the location of the sound.

Breath sounds are identified by their intensity, their pitch, and the relative duration of their inspiratory and expiratory phases.

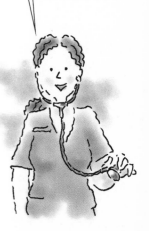

Normal breath sounds vary significantly, depending on the auscultation site.

Listening to normal breath sounds

During auscultation, you'll notice a marked difference in normal breath sounds, depending on where you auscultate. For example, large airways such as the trachea have turbulent airflow, producing loud breath sounds. However, as the air travels throughout the airways and past the segmental bronchi, the airflow pattern changes. Furthermore, the chest wall, pleurae, and air-filled tissue filter the sounds, causing them to diminish. That's why normal breath sounds, heard over most of the chest wall, are soft and low-pitched.

Mouth too mouth

Normal breath sounds include tracheal, bronchial, vesicular, and bronchovesicular sounds as well as the sounds heard at the patient's mouth.

Tracheal and bronchial breath sounds

Turbulent airflow patterns produce the breath sounds normally heard over the trachea (tracheal breath sounds **(1)**) and mainstem bronchi (bronchial breath sounds **(7, 8)**). (See *Locating tracheal and bronchial breath sounds*.)

That sounds harsh!

Both tracheal and bronchial breath sounds are high-pitched, although the pitch may change, depending on the auscultation site. Tracheal breath sounds are harsh; you'll hear them best over the trachea and larynx. Bronchial breath sounds are loud; you'll hear them next to the tra-

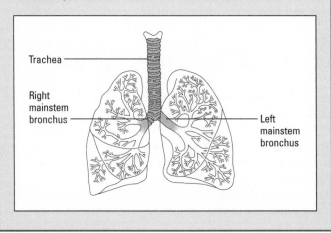

Locating tracheal and bronchial breath sounds

The highlighted portions of this illustration of the lungs show the areas that produce tracheal and bronchial breath sounds.

Trachea

Right mainstem bronchus

Left mainstem bronchus

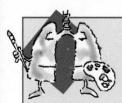

Inspired work

Auscultation sites for tracheal and bronchial breath sounds

To hear tracheal and bronchial breath sounds, auscultate the patient's chest on either side of the sternum from the second to the fourth intercostal space and the patient's back along the vertebral column from the third to the sixth intercostal space, as highlighted in the illustrations below.

Anterior view

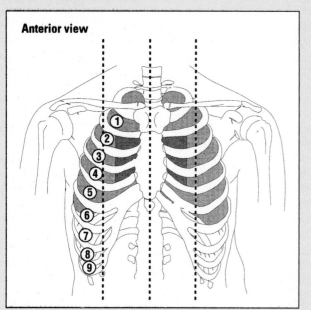

Posterior view

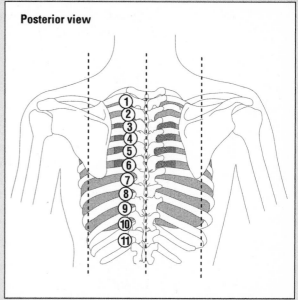

chea and larynx. Use the diaphragm of a stethoscope to auscultate these sounds.

You'll hear these sounds throughout inspiration and expiration, although the sound lasts longer on expiration. **(7, 8)** You may also notice that the sound pauses briefly at the end of inspiration. Specifically, the inspiratory-expiratory (I:E) ratio of tracheal and bronchial breath sounds is 1:2 to 1:3, and the sound frequency distribution is 200 to 2,000 hertz. **(7, 8)** (See *Auscultation sites for tracheal and bronchial breath sounds.*)

Vesicular breath sounds

Transmitted through lung tissue and the chest wall, vesicular breath sounds result from changes in airflow patterns. You'll hear them throughout the chest (except over the upper sternum and between the scapulae), although they're most audible over the bases of the lungs. (See *Locating vesicular breath sounds.*)

Soft spoken

These normal sounds are quieter than tracheal and bronchial sounds, have a low pitch, and make a "swishing" sound. Clearly audible on inspiration, the sounds have a long inspiratory phase, but quickly fade on expiration as airflow rates rapidly decline and turbulent airflow moves toward the central airways. The I:E ratio for vesicular breath sounds is 3:1 to 4:1. **(9, 10, 11)** (See *Auscultation sites for vesicular breath sounds.*)

> Turbulent air makes for a bumpy flight AND loud breath sounds!

Locating vesicular breath sounds

The highlighted portions of this illustration show the airway areas that produce vesicular breath sounds.

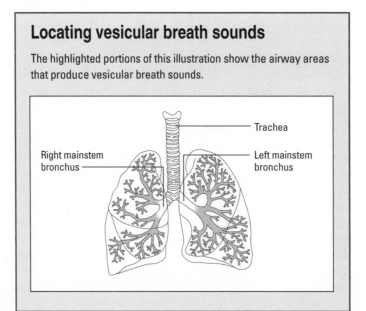

Trachea

Right mainstem bronchus

Left mainstem bronchus

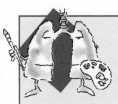

Inspired work

Auscultation sites for vesicular breath sounds

The highlighted areas on these illustrations show the best sites for auscultating vesicular breath sounds over the patient's chest and back. Keep in mind that the sounds will be loudest over the lung bases.

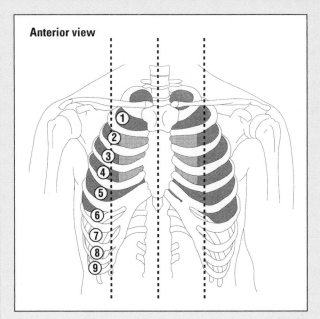

Anterior view

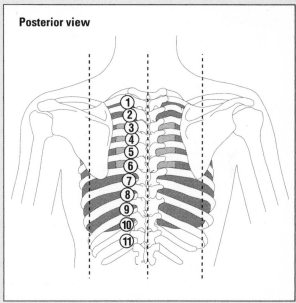

Posterior view

Bronchovesicular breath sounds

When auscultating over the large airways, both anteriorly and posteriorly, you'll normally hear bronchovesicular breath sounds. The pitch and duration of these sounds is midway between that of vesicular and bronchial breath sounds. The inspiratory and expiratory phases of bronchovesicular breath sounds are equal, with an I:E ratio of 1:1. (See *Auscultation sites for bronchovesicular breath sounds*, page 64.)

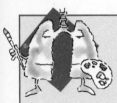

Inspired work

Auscultation sites for bronchovesicular breath sounds

To hear bronchovesicular breath sounds the best, listen to the patient's chest at the first and second intercostal spaces or to his back between the scapulae, as highlighted in the illustrations below.

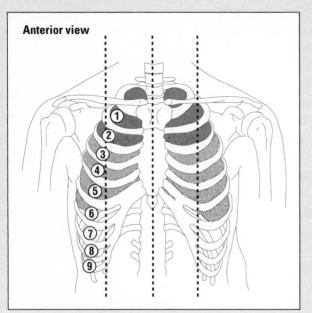

Anterior view

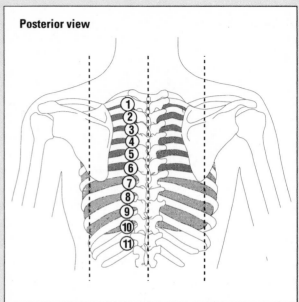

Posterior view

Breath sounds at the mouth

You can also hear normal breath sounds when you listen near the patient's lips. Most likely produced by turbulent airflow below the glottis and before the terminal airways, these breath sounds provide a baseline that can be used later to evaluate noisy or paradoxically quiet breath sounds.

Mouthing off

The intensity of these breath sounds is as loud and harsh as that of tracheal and bronchial breath sounds. The sounds, which have a moderately high pitch, persist throughout the respiratory cycle.

Evaluating bronchovesicular breath sounds

The intensity of bronchovesicular breath sounds normally changes during deep inspiration and after maximal expiration. These variations typically result from airflow patterns and the distribution of ventilation through the lungs, although variations in intensity may also occur between regions of the lung.

Changes during the respiratory cycle

When auscultating the chest of a patient who's sitting up, you'll notice that bronchovesicular breath sounds are louder over the apices of the lungs during early inspiration and become progressively softer as inspiration continues. **(10)** That's because, when the patient inhales while in an upright position, air flows into the lung apices first before flowing into the lung bases, which are in a dependent position.

Gaining momentum

If you then listen at the patient's back over the lung bases, you'll notice that bronchovesicular breath sounds are initially soft and grow progressively louder with maximal inspiration. You may not notice these changes, however, unless you ask the patient to take deep breaths.

Remember that exaggerated breathing can be tiring for young, elderly, and ill patients. Be alert for lightheadedness or faintness related to hyperventilation from deep breathing. Allow the patient rest periods as needed.

Lungs fill with air from the top down. That's why breath sounds are loudest in the apices at the beginning of inspiration and loudest in the bases at the end.

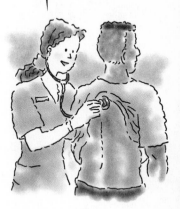

Changes with the cardiac cycle

Breath sounds heard over the left lower lobe may also vary in intensity during the cardiac cycle.

Room to grow

During systole, when the ventricle contracts, the surrounding lung tissue has room to expand more fully. This increases turbulent airflow to that region and intensifies inspiratory sounds.

Cramped for space

On the other hand, during diastole, the expanding ventricle compresses adjacent lung tissue and reduces airflow to that region, which decreases intensity.

Bronchovesicular breath sounds are heard throughout the chest anteriorly, posteriorly, and laterally. Their duration varies, depending on their location, but inspiration is usually followed immediately by a shorter expiration. These sounds have a low pitch that can be heard with either the diaphragm or bell of the stethoscope. **(11)**

Hey! Stop crowding my space!

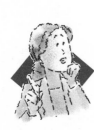

Quick quiz

1. Normal breath sounds heard over most of the chest wall are described as being:
    A.   loud.
    B.   high-pitched.
    C.   rumbling.
    D.   soft.

Answer: D. Normal breath sounds heard over most of the chest wall surface are soft and low-pitched; they're softer and shorter during expiration than during inspiration.

2. Tracheal and bronchial breath sounds are heard:
    A.   anteriorly, from the second to the fourth intercostal space.
    B.   posteriorly, from the first to the sixth intercostal space.
    C.   posteriorly, along the eighth and ninth intercostal spaces.
    D.   over most of the anterior chest wall.

Answer: A. Tracheal and bronchial breath sounds are heard over the chest wall on either side of the sternum from the second to the fourth intercostal space. Posteriorly, they're heard along the vertebral column from the third to the sixth intercostal space.

3. Vesicular breath sounds:
   A. are louder than tracheal or bronchial breath sounds.
   B. are more sibilant than tracheal or bronchial breath sounds.
   C. are quieter than tracheal or bronchial breath sounds.
   D. sound similar to tracheal and bronchial breath sounds.

Answer: C. Vesicular sounds are quieter than tracheal or bronchial sounds, which are loud due to the turbulent airflow pattern and are usually high-pitched. Vesicular breath sounds also usually have a low pitch compared with tracheal and bronchial sounds.

4. Normal breath sounds audible at the mouth are heard:
   A. near the trachea.
   B. at the lips.
   C. at the same sites as vesicular breath sounds.
   D. over the chest wall.

Answer: B. Normal breath sounds audible at the mouth are heard at the lips and can provide a baseline that can be used to evaluate noisy or paradoxically quiet breath sounds.

5. During the cardiac cycle, breath sounds heard over which part of the lungs vary in intensity?
   A. Left lower lobe
   B. Right lower lobe
   C. Left anterior apex
   D. Right anterior apex

Answer: A. Breath sounds heard over the left lower lobe may vary in intensity during the cardiac cycle. During systole, inspiratory sounds intensify due to ventricular contraction and lung expansion. During diastole, sound intensity decreases as the ventricle dilates and compresses lung tissue.

Scoring

☆☆☆ If you answered all five questions correctly, stupendous! Your comprehension of normal breath sounds is breathtaking!

☆☆ If you answered four questions correctly, way to go! You can breathe easy now that you have a handle on normal breath sounds.

☆ If you answered fewer than four questions correctly, don't worry. Take a minute to catch your breath and then take the quiz again.

Bronchial breath sounds

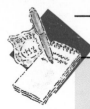

Just the facts

In this chapter, you'll learn:
♦ characteristics of bronchial breath sounds
♦ the effect of increased lung density on normal breath sounds
♦ specific conditions affecting breath sounds.

Bronchial breath sounds at a glance

Bronchial breath sounds are loud, high-pitched sounds that have a hollow or harsh quality. They're normally heard next to the trachea. Bronchial breath sounds are considered abnormal when found anywhere except anteriorly over the large airways.

Abnormal bronchial breath sounds

Bronchial breath sounds occur in abnormal areas when lung tissue between the central airways and the chest wall becomes airless from increased lung density.

Full speed ahead

The dense lung tissue creates an impedance match between itself, the pleurae, and the chest wall. Consequently, sound travels more readily to the chest wall, and the normal filtering of high-frequency sounds fails to occur. The resulting breath sounds are louder and more tubular than normal breath sounds heard over the same area. Also, expiration is significantly louder and longer than normal. The inspiratory-expiratory (I:E) ratio changes from the normal 3:1 or 4:1 to 1:1 or 1:2.

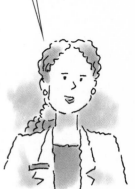

Remember, bronchial breath sounds are an abnormal finding when they occur anywhere other than anteriorly over the large airways.

Conditions causing bronchial breath sounds

Conditions associated with bronchial breath sounds include consolidation, atelectasis, and fibrosis, all of which increase lung tissue density because of fluid accumulation, lung collapse, or fibrotic scarring. Bronchial breath sounds occur over the affected lung area.

Consolidation

In consolidation (solidification), fluid, leukocytes, and erythrocytes accumulate in spaces that are normally air-filled, producing a consolidated area. Clinical findings vary, depending on the location of the consolidated area and the causative agent.

The most common cause of lung tissue consolidation is pneumonia, a lung inflammation that can be caused by bacteria, viruses, or chemical insults (such as with aspiration).

Patent-cy pending

With classic consolidation, you'll note decreased chest wall movement and dullness to percussion over the affected area. You'll also hear bronchial breath sounds over a dense, airless *upper* lobe, even without a patent bronchus. **(12, 13)** That's because the upper lobe surfaces contact the trachea, and loud tracheal breath sounds travel directly to the dense, airless upper lobe tissues. In contrast, you'll only hear bronchial breath sounds over a dense, airless *lower* lobe when the bronchi are patent. That's because sound doesn't travel directly to the airless lower lobe tissues.

What you hear

In a patient with lobar pneumonia and right posterior midlung consolidation, you'll hear bronchial breath sounds over the right posterior midlung field. This area is located over the seventh and eighth intercostal spaces along the

Your percussion sounds really dull today. Do you feel all right?

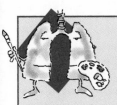

Inspired work

Bronchial breath sounds in consolidated lung tissue

The highlighted areas in these illustrations show the location of bronchial breath sounds in a patient with consolidation in the middle of the right lung.

Affected lung area

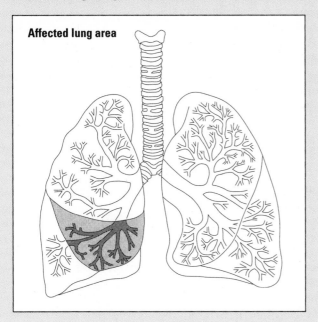

Posterior auscultatory sites

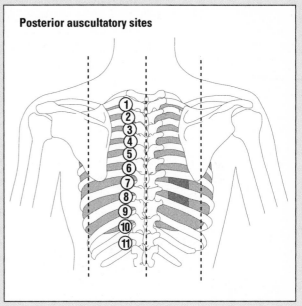

vertebral column. (See *Bronchial breath sounds in consolidated lung tissue.*)

Hear for the duration

These sounds are high-pitched and have the typical hollow, or tubular, quality of normal central airway breath sounds. They remain audible during both expiration and inspiration, but the expiratory sounds are longer and louder when the patient is sitting up; the I:E ratio is 1:2. These sounds may be auscultated with either the bell or diaphragm of the stethoscope. **(12, 13)**

Atelectasis

Atelectasis, incomplete expansion of a lung area, is typically diagnosed in postoperative or immobile patients and in some patients with bronchiectasis or pneumonia.

Lack of use

Atelectasis is thought to result from prolonged shallow breathing (hypoventilation) or uncleared secretions that occlude the airway. Because no air enters the distal airways, the segmental or lobar bronchi collapse. If a large airway is occluded, clinical findings include decreased chest wall movement, a dull percussion note, regional changes in lung volume, and bronchial breath sounds over a dense, airless upper airway. **(14, 15)** (See *Bronchial breath sounds in atelectasis.*)

Decreased chest wall movement and lung volume changes may be difficult to detect on examination. If you hear bronchial breath sounds in upper lobes and absent breath sounds in lower lobes, assume a large airway occlusion is present. Be sure to implement measures to maintain oxygenation and a patent airway.

What you hear

You'll hear bronchial breath sounds over an atelectatic area when the bronchus is patent. You won't hear them over an atelectatic lower lobe if the bronchus is obstructed.

Right in the middle

In an unresponsive patient, you'll hear bronchial breath sounds over the right anterior midlung field, located between the third and fifth intercostal spaces from the midsternal line to just right of the midclavicular line. These sounds are high-pitched and have the typical hollow, or tubular, quality of normal central airway breath sounds. They're audible throughout inspiration and expiration. When the patient is in the supine position, the inspiratory and expiratory sounds are equal in duration and intensity; the I:E ratio is 1:1. These sounds can be heard equally well with either the bell or diaphragm of the stethoscope. **(14, 15)**

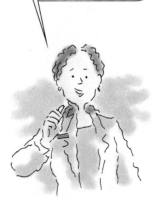

Be alert! If you detect bronchial breath sounds in the patient's upper lobes and absent breath sounds in the lower lobes, suspect a large airway occlusion. Take immediate steps to ensure adequate oxygenation.

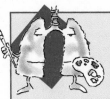

Inspired work

Bronchial breath sounds in atelectasis

Use these illustrations to guide you when auscultating a patient with atelectasis in the right midlung region. The highlighted areas show where you'll most likely hear bronchial breath sounds.

Affected lung area

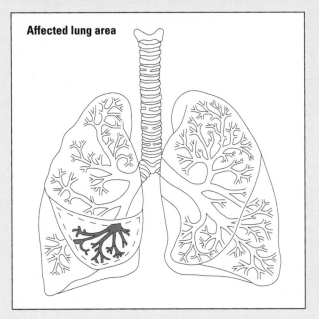

Anterior auscultatory sites

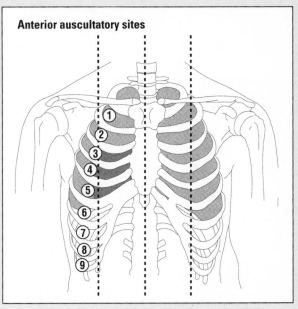

Fibrosis

Severe fibrosis (abnormal formation of fibrous connective tissue) may produce bronchial breath sounds that are usually heard over the lower lung regions. Interstitial pulmonary fibrosis is a pathologic change caused by many chronic inflammatory diseases that produce diffuse lung injury.

Another reason not to smoke!

Some possible causes of pulmonary fibrosis include chronic smoke inhalation and chronic exposure to asbestos. In most cases, however, the cause is unknown. The breath sounds

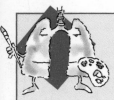

Inspired work

Bronchial breath sounds in asbestosis

These illustrations highlight the areas where you'll most likely hear bronchial breath sounds in a patient with asbestosis.

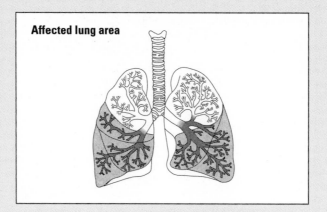

Affected lung area

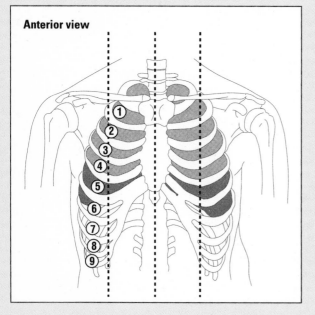

Anterior view

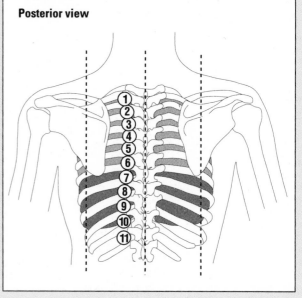

Posterior view

heard over fibrotic areas are similar to those heard over atelectatic areas. **(16, 17)**

What you hear

In some patients with asbestosis, bronchial breath sounds are heard anteriorly and posteriorly over both lung bases. Anteriorly, this area extends from the midsternal line to the right and left of the anterior axillary lines over the fifth and sixth intercostal spaces; posteriorly, it extends from the vertebral line to the right and left of the posterior axillary lines over the seventh, eighth, ninth, and tenth intercostal spaces. (See *Bronchial breath sounds in asbestosis*.)

Because the bronchi are patent, bronchial breath sounds heard over fibrotic areas have the typical hollow, or tubular, quality of normal central airway breath sounds. You'll hear them throughout inspiration and expiration.

Don't be so loud

When the patient is in the upright position, the breath sounds become progressively louder during inspiration and become both louder and longer during expiration; the I:E ratio is 1:1 to 1:2. These bronchial breath sounds are high-pitched and are heard equally well with either the diaphragm or bell of the stethoscope. **(16, 17)**

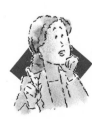

Quick quiz

1. The most common cause of lung tissue consolidation is:

    A.   pleurisy.
    B.   varicella.
    C.   pneumonia.
    D.   influenza.

Answer: C. The most common cause of lung tissue consolidation is pneumonia, a lung inflammation that can be caused by bacteria, viruses, or chemical insults (such as with aspiration).

2.   If you hear bronchial breath sounds in the upper lobes and absent breath sounds in lower lobes, you should:
    A.   document these normal findings in the medical record.
    B.   encourage the patient to ambulate.
    C.   agree to the patient's request to remove his nasal oxygen cannula.
    D.   provide measures to maintain oxygenation and a patent airway.

Answer: D. If you hear bronchial breath sounds in the upper lobes and absent breath sounds in the lower lobes, assume a large airway occlusion is present. You should implement measures to maintain oxygenation and a patent airway.

3.   Atelectasis is defined as:
    A.   incomplete expansion of a lung area.
    B.   consolidation of lung tissue.
    C.   abnormal formation of fibrous tissue.
    D.   pulmonary fibrosis.

Answer: A. Atelectasis is incomplete expansion of a lung area.

4.   One possible cause of pulmonary fibrosis is:
    A.   pneumonia.
    B.   chronic smoke inhalation.
    C.   prolonged shallow breathing.
    D.   immobility.

Answer: B. Chronic smoke inhalation is a possible cause of pulmonary fibrosis.

Scoring

☆☆☆ If you answered all four questions correctly, congratulations! You've braved bronchial breath sounds and won!

☆☆ If you answered three questions correctly, excellent work! Sounds like you've mastered these abnormal sounds!

☆ If you answered fewer than three questions correctly, don't despair. Take a break from these breath sounds and then try the quick quiz again.

Abnormal voice sounds

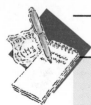

Just the facts

In this chapter, you'll learn:

♦ the origin of normal voice sounds

♦ three types of abnormally transmitted voice sounds

♦ auscultatory findings associated with consolidation.

Voice sounds at a glance

Voice sounds are vibrations produced by speech that are transmitted to the chest wall through the tracheobronchial tree. Abnormal transmission of voice sounds typically occurs over consolidated areas of lung tissue (areas that have solidified due to inflammation or tumors). Therefore, voice sounds heard during an auscultatory assessment provide valuable clues about the condition of the patient's lungs.

Sounds normal

Voice sounds result when air from the lungs passes over the vocal cords, producing vibrations. In turn, the resonance of the mouth, nasopharynx, and paranasal sinuses amplifies these sounds. Healthy, air-filled lungs normally filter high-frequency sounds such as vowel sounds. The pleurae also reflect voice sounds back toward the lung tissue, further diminishing the sounds. Therefore, when you auscultate healthy lungs, transmitted voice sounds should sound like low-pitched, unintelligible mumbles.

Sound off!

On the other hand, consolidated or atelectatic lung tissue enhances sound transmission. When you auscultate lungs with one of these conditions, voice sounds are more distinct.

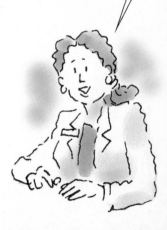

When you auscultate over normal lung tissue, voice sounds are unintelligible. It's only over areas of consolidation or atelectasis that the sounds become distinct.

Types of abnormal voice sounds

The three types of abnormally transmitted voice sounds are bronchophony, whispered pectoriloquy, and egophony.

Bronchophony

When voice sounds are heard clearly and distinctly during auscultation, this is called *bronchophony*. **(18)** Occurring over dense, airless lung tissue, bronchophony results from impedance matching, which causes high-frequency vowel sounds to travel more easily to the chest wall. Consolidation also increases vocal resonance, which further allows the clear transmission of voice sounds to the chest wall.

Taking the direct route

For bronchophony to occur, a direct path for sound transmission must exist. For example, you'll hear bronchophony over dense, airless upper lobes because the surface of the lung's upper lobes has direct contact with the trachea. This allows tracheal breath sounds to travel directly to the chest wall. In contrast, for bronchophony to occur over dense, airless lower lobes, the bronchi must be patent, or open. Otherwise, there's no direct path for sound transmission.

What you hear

You'll most commonly hear bronchophony over consolidated areas of lung tissue in the upper lobes. Bronchophony may occur anywhere over the anterior, lateral, or posterior chest wall surfaces. (See *Consolidation in the left upper lobe.*)

To check for bronchophony, ask the patient to say "ninety-nine" several times. Over healthy lung tissue, the words sound unintelligible. **(19)** Over consolidated areas, the high-frequency sounds are easily understood as words. **(20)** (See *Auscultating for bronchophony in left upper lobe pneumonia*, page 80.)

Memory jogger

To remember how the direct path of sound transmission occurs in bronchophony, think **BUD** but **BLOP**:

Bronchophony

Upper lobes

Direct contact with trachea

but

Bronchophony

LOwer lobes

Patent bronchi.

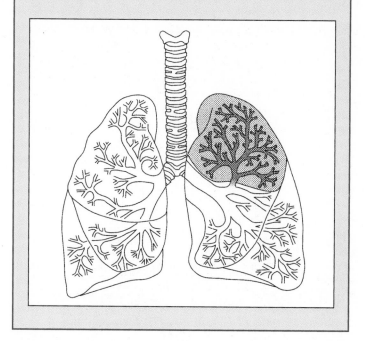

Consolidation in the left upper lobe

This illustration highlights a consolidated lung area in the left upper lobe. On auscultation, you would typically hear bronchophony in this area.

Whispered pectoriloquy

The clear, distinct, whispered voice sound transmitted through airless, consolidated, or atelectatic lung tissue is known as *whispered pectoriloquy*.

Sotto voce

In a healthy person, normal lung tissue filters the high-frequency sounds of whispered vowels, making them unintelligible during auscultation. In a patient with consolidation or atelectasis, whispered vowel sounds travel to the chest wall without much filtering, making them audible during auscultation. **(21)**

What you hear

You can hear whispered pectoriloquy over areas of dense, airless lung tissue, such as from consolidation or atelecta-

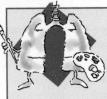

Inspired work

Auscultating for bronchophony in left upper lobe pneumonia

In a patient with left upper lobe pneumonia, which results in consolidation, you'll auscultate intelligible voice sounds over both the anterior and posterior chest wall surfaces. To auscultate the anterior chest wall, listen over the area from just above the clavicle down to the second intercostal space and from the midsternal line to the left of the midclavicular line. To auscultate the posterior area, listen between the first and third intercostal spaces from the vertebral line toward the left midscapular line.

Anterior view

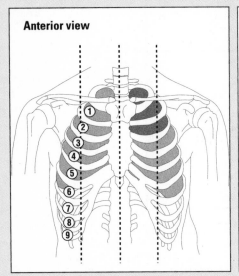

Posterior view

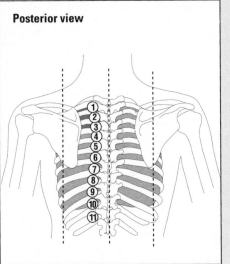

sis. You may hear this voice sound anywhere over the anterior or posterior chest wall surface. (*See Atelectasis in the left lower lobe.*)

Whisper down the lane

During auscultation, ask the patient to whisper the words "one, two, three" several times. Over healthy lung tissue, the words sound unintelligible. **(22)** However, over an area of atelectasis, the high-frequency vowel sounds are easily understood as words. **(23)**

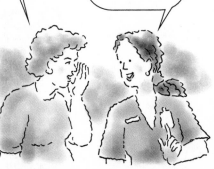

Atelectasis in the left lower lobe

This illustration shows an area of atelectasis in the left lower lobe. An area such as this would produce whispered pectoriloquy.

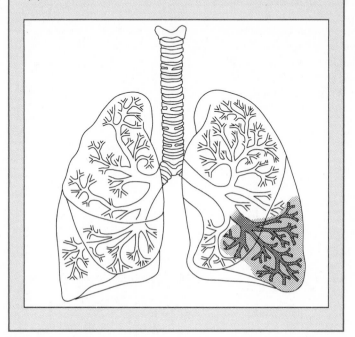

(See *Auscultating for whispered pectoriloquy in left lower lobe atelectasis*, page 82.)

Egophony

Because impedance matching enhances the transmission of breath sounds over areas of consolidation or atelectasis, voice sounds may have a nasal or bleating quality when heard over the chest wall. **(24)** This is called *egophony*. Egophony may also occur at the upper edge of a large pleural effusion. (See *Consolidation in the right lower lobe*, page 83.)

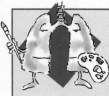

Inspired work

Auscultating for whispered pectoriloquy in left lower lobe atelectasis

When auscultating the lungs of a patient with left lower lobe atelectasis and a patent bronchus, you'll hear voice sounds over the anterior and posterior chest wall surfaces. To auscultate the anterior area, listen over the fifth and sixth intercostal spaces from the midsternal line to the midaxillary line. To auscultate the posterior area, listen over the eighth, ninth, and tenth intercostal spaces from the vertebral line to the midaxillary line.

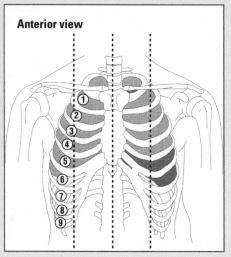

Anterior view

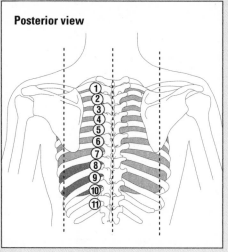

Posterior view

What you hear

You'll hear egophony over a consolidated or atelectatic area on the anterior, posterior, or lateral chest wall surface. (See *Auscultating for egophony in right lower lobe pneumonia*, page 84.)

To detect egophony, ask the patient to repeat the letter "E" several times. Over healthy lung tissue, you'll hear a normal sounding "E." **(25)** Over consolidated areas, you'll hear a high-pitched sound with a nasal quality, sounding like "A." **(26)**

Memory jogger

To remember the proper words to use during your assessment for abnormal breath sounds as well as how these words should sound, remember these three quips:

• Bronchophony makes "ninety-nine" sound just fine.

• Whispered pectoriloquy equals clear as can be "1, 2, 3."

• Egophony causes you to hear an "A" rather than an "E."

Consolidation in the right lower lobe

This illustration shows a consolidated area in the right lower lobe of the lung. An area such as this would produce egophony.

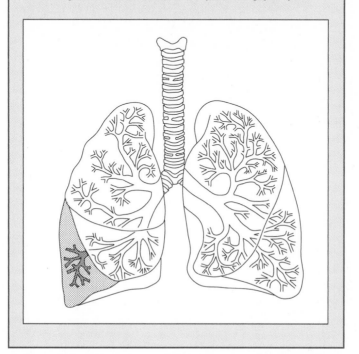

Understanding abnormal voice sounds

It's important to know that a constellation of auscultatory findings — bronchial breath sounds, bronchophony, whispered pectoriloquy, and egophony — typically occurs in patients with consolidation. Bronchophony may be easier to hear in patients with pronounced bronchial breath sounds who have consolidation in a single lobe or lung. Whispered pectoriloquy is typically discernible over atelectatic lung segments or areas of patchy consolidation where bronchial sounds or bronchophony isn't completely audible.

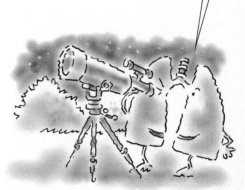

A constellation of auscultatory findings occurs in patients with consolidation.

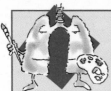

Inspired work

Auscultating for egophony in right lower lobe pneumonia

In a patient with right lower lobe pneumonia, you'll hear egophony when auscultating the lateral chest wall surface. Specifically, listen over the fifth and sixth intercostal spaces between the anterior axillary line and the midaxillary line.

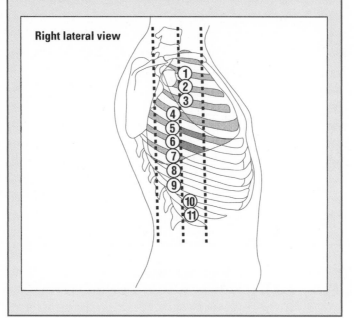

Right lateral view

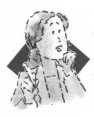

Quick quiz

1. Voice sounds result from:
    A. air passing through the paranasal sinuses.
    B. spasm of the nasopharynx.
    C. vibrations of the vocal cords.
    D. sound waves against the upper palate of the mouth.

Answer: C. Voice sounds result from vibrations of the vocal cords as air from the lungs passes over them.

2. To detect changes in bronchophony, you should ask the patient to repeat the:
- A. letter "E."
- B. words "one, two, three."
- C. vowels "a, e, i, o, u."
- D. word "ninety-nine."

Answer: D. To detect changes in bronchophony, ask the patient to repeat the word "ninety-nine" several times. Over healthy lung tissue, the words sound unintelligible; over a consolidated area, the high-frequency sounds are easily understood.

3. Over dense, airless lung tissue whispered pectoriloquy:
- A. sounds garbled.
- B. is audible without a stethoscope.
- C. produces a clear, distinct, intelligible whispered voice sound.
- D. sounds muffled and difficult to hear.

Answer: C. Whispered pectoriloquy produces a clear, distinct, intelligible, whispered voice sound over airless, consolidated, or atelectatic lung tissue.

4. Egophony can be described as:
- A. a voice sound with a nasal or bleating quality when heard over the chest wall.
- B. unintelligible transmission of the word "ninety-nine."
- C. a wheezing sound heard on inspiration.
- D. the clear transmission of whispered high-frequency vowel sounds.

Answer: A. Egophony is a voice sound that has a nasal or bleating quality when heard over the chest wall.

5. When voice sounds pass through normally inflated, air-filled lungs, vowel tones are:
- A. distinct.
- B. amplified.
- C. diminished and filtered.
- D. clarified and less filtered.

Answer: C. When voice sounds pass through normally inflated, air-filled lungs, vowel tones are diminished and filtered.

Scoring

☆☆☆ If you answered all five questions correctly, shout with joy! We'll proclaim your mastery of abnormal voice sounds as loud as we can!

☆☆ If you answered four questions correctly, feel free to sing your own praises! We'll echo a job well done!

☆ If you answered fewer than four questions correctly, don't feel you have to keep quiet. A little more study, and you'll be speaking up about voice sounds in no time.

Absent and diminished breath sounds

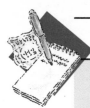

Just the facts

In this chapter, you'll learn:

♦ conditions associated with diminished or absent breath sounds

♦ the ways in which specific conditions cause diminished or absent breath sounds

♦ effects of impedance mismatch and filtering on sound transmission.

Absent and diminished breath sounds at a glance

Any condition that limits the flow of air into the lungs causes breath sounds to become diminished or absent. If the flow rate of inspired air slows, less air movement occurs. In turn, airflow becomes less turbulent, and the amplitude of breath sounds diminishes.

Feeling incompatible

Diminished or absent breath sounds can also be caused by an impedance mismatch — a condition that occurs when sound travels through two substances that have significantly different acoustic properties. When this occurs, sound transmission is filtered or altered. An example of an impedance mismatch is when sound passes from an air-filled area of lung tissue through a collection of fluid. Sound may also be diminished from increased chest wall thickness, such as occurs in obesity.

Diminished breath sounds result from any condition that limits airflow into the lungs or from a lung condition that disrupts the transmission of breath sounds.

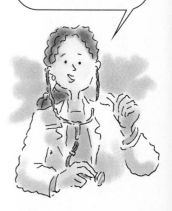

Conditions causing absent and diminished breath sounds

As previously stated, any condition that limits airflow into the lungs can diminish or eliminate breath sounds. Such conditions include shallow breathing, diaphragmatic paralysis, severe airway obstruction, pneumothorax, hemothorax, pleural effusion, hyperinflated lungs, and obesity. The use of positive end-expiratory pressure (PEEP) during mechanical ventilation may also contribute to diminished breath sounds.

Shallow breathing

When a person breathes normally while in an upright position, most of the respiratory movement—and, therefore, most of the ventilation—occurs in the dependent regions of the lungs.

Don't be so shallow

During shallow breathing, less respiratory movement occurs. Consequently, airflow decreases, resulting in decreased turbulence and, therefore, diminished breath sounds. **(27)** (See *A look at decreased turbulence.*)

What you hear

You'll hear diminished, softer sounds caused by shallow breathing over the anterior, posterior, and lateral chest wall surfaces. Postoperative patients and patients with rib fractures commonly breathe shallowly because pain limits their depth of respiration. Patients with decreased levels of consciousness from central nervous system injuries or drug overdoses may also have shallow breathing.

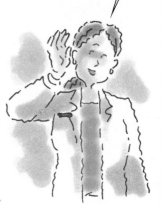

You'll hear diminished, softer sounds in a patient with shallow breathing.

Diaphragmatic paralysis

During inspiration, the dome-shaped diaphragm contracts, expanding the lower rib cage, forcing the abdominal contents downward and out, and increasing the length of the lungs. This process lowers intrapulmonary pressure and allows air to flow into the airways.

Breathe easy

A look at decreased turbulence

When breathing becomes shallow, air turbulence decreases. As a result, breath sounds are diminished. These illustrations show the change in turbulence that occurs with shallow breathing.

Normal turbulent airflow

Airway walls

Decreased turbulent airflow in shallow breathing

Airway walls

Second in command

If the diaphragm becomes paralyzed, which may occur after injury to the phrenic nerve, it can no longer participate in normal breathing. The internal and external intercostal muscles, which have a supportive role in normal breathing, must assume control. With only these chest wall muscles initiating the respiratory cycle, ventilation of the lung bases may be limited, resulting in diminished breath sounds.

Ever since the diaphragm quit working, my bases never seem to get a good workout.

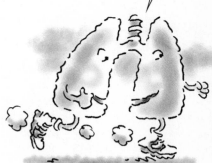

What you hear

You'll hear diminished sounds caused by diaphragmatic paralysis over the anterior, posterior, and lateral chest wall surfaces. **(28)** When caring for a patient with diaphragmatic paralysis and greatly diminished breath sounds, be alert for signs of respiratory distress. Prepare for intubation and mechanical ventilation as necessary.

> Diaphragmatic paralysis may cause respiratory distress, possibly necessitating intubation or mechanical ventilation.

Airway obstruction

An obstruction in an airway blocks the flow of air and, therefore, changes the breath sounds heard during auscultation. The location of the obstruction determines where you'll hear the changes in breath sounds.

What you hear

If a lobar or segmental bronchus becomes obstructed from, for example, a foreign object or a large mucus plug, airflow stops distal to the obstruction. As a result, breath sounds are absent over the area distal to the obstruction. (See *Lobar bronchus obstruction.*)

If a mainstem bronchus becomes obstructed, breath sounds are absent throughout the entire affected lung. (See *Mainstem bronchus obstruction,* page 92.)

Path of least resistance

Because the right mainstem bronchus extends from the trachea in a straight line, aspirated foreign bodies are more likely to lodge there. Likewise, endotracheal tubes are frequently misplaced in the right mainstem bronchus. If breath sounds are absent throughout the right lung field after intubation, the endotracheal tube should be repositioned and breath sounds reevaluated.

Pneumothorax

Pneumothorax occurs when a tear in the visceral or parietal pleura allows air to accumulate in the normally airless pleural space. An impedance mismatch occurs between the air-filled lung and the collection of air in the pleural space. This causes breath sounds to be significantly diminished or absent over the area of pneumothorax. **(29)**

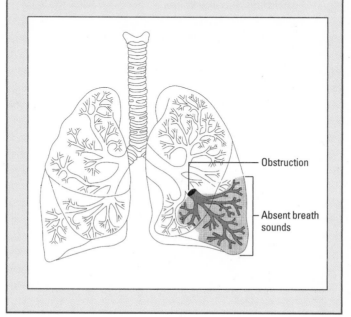

Lobar bronchus obstruction

Conditions that limit airflow into lung segments—such as a severe airway obstruction—can diminish or even eliminate breath sounds. This illustration shows a lobar bronchus obstruction along with the area in which breath sounds would be absent.

A tense situation

In *uncomplicated pneumothorax*, air enters and leaves the pleural space easily. In certain instances, however, air enters the pleural space with every breath and becomes trapped. This is known as *tension pneumothorax*.

Collapsing under pressure

As the trapped air accumulates, it exerts pressure on the lung, causing it to collapse. The increasing pressure may shift the mediastinum to the opposite side, causing decreased cardiac output. Unless the intrapleural air is evacuated immediately, this condition may become life threatening, particularly if the patient is being ventilated mechanically.

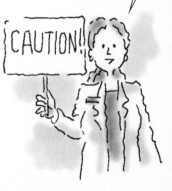

Patients being mechanically ventilated are at risk for developing life-threatening tension pneumothorax. That's because the ventilator continues to supply air at a fixed flow rate and pressure even after pneumothorax develops.

Mainstem bronchus obstruction

An obstruction in the main bronchus stops the flow of air to the entire lung, causing breath sounds to become absent.

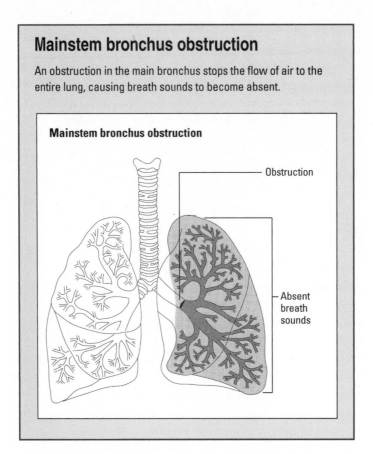

Mainstem bronchus obstruction

Obstruction

Absent breath sounds

Signs and symptoms of pneumothorax include sharp, stabbing chest pain; dyspnea; absent breath sounds; inaudible egophony, bronchophony, and whispered pectoriloquy; and increased resonance during percussion. Tension pneumothorax may cause decreased cardiac output, hypotension, and eventually death.

What you hear

Diminished or absent breath sounds resulting from pneumothorax can be heard anywhere over the anterior, posterior, and lateral chest wall surfaces, depending on the location and size of the pneumothorax.

Feeling overlooked

A small pneumothorax, which may be visible on a chest X-ray, may not alter breath sound intensity enough to be

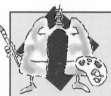

Inspired work

Pneumothorax of the left lung

The illustration below left shows pneumothorax in the left lateral lung field, which can be auscultated over the fourth, fifth, sixth, and seventh intercostal spaces between the anterior and posterior axillary folds (highlighted in the illustration below right). When this occurs, you can hear normal breath sounds on the contralateral side over healthy lung tissue. **(30)** Breath sounds are absent over the area of pneumothorax. **(31)** Any diminished breath sounds have a low pitch that's heard best with either the bell or diaphragm of the stethoscope.

Pneumothorax affecting left lateral lung field

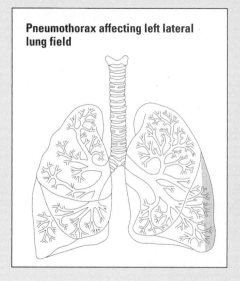

Left lateral auscultatory sites

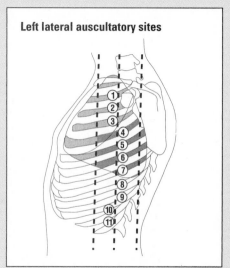

heard during auscultation. A large pneumothorax significantly diminishes or blocks breath sounds. (See *Pneumothorax of the left lung.*)

Pleural effusion

Pleural effusion is the accumulation of fluid in the pleural space. This condition creates an impedance mismatch that causes diminished or absent breath sounds. **(32)** (See *Pleural effusion in the right lower lobe,* page 94.)

A large pleural effusion compresses adjacent lung tissue, causing atelectasis and producing a dull percussion

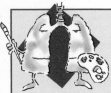

Inspired work

Pleural effusion in the right lower lobe

The illustration below left shows pleural effusion in the right lower lung. When this occurs, you can hear diminished breath sounds over the eighth, ninth, and tenth intercostal spaces (highlighted in the illustration below right), from the vertebral line just to the right of the midscapular line. You can hear normal breath sounds on the contralateral side over healthy lung tissue. **(33)** The diminished breath sounds have a low pitch that's heard best with either the bell or diaphragm of the stethoscope. **(34)**

Affected lung area

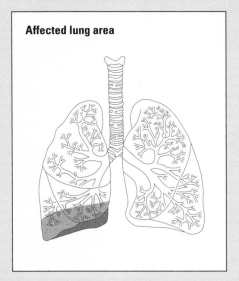

Posterior auscultatory sites

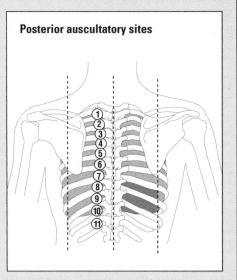

tone. You may detect egophony, bronchophony, and whispered pectoriloquy at the upper border of the pleural effusion.

What you hear

Diminished or absent breath sounds resulting from pleural effusion may be heard anywhere over the anterior, posterior, or lateral chest wall surfaces, depending on pleural effusion location. If pleural effusion is large, you'll also note diminished or absent sounds over the lower right anterior and lateral chest wall surfaces.

An intense personality

Occasionally, very loud bronchial breath sounds have enough intensity to travel through a small pleural effusion. Be sure to monitor a patient with a pleural effusion for respiratory distress. Prepare for chest tube insertion, if necessary.

Hyperinflated lungs

When a lung becomes hyperinflated, it compresses the large central airways. The lung also loses elastic tension, and the airways may have an increased resistance to airflow. These factors limit airflow during expiration, causing decreased breath sounds. (See *A close look at hyperinflated alveoli.*)

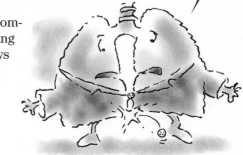

Oh, boy. I'm so puffed up that I'm compressing my central airways and none of my clothes fit!

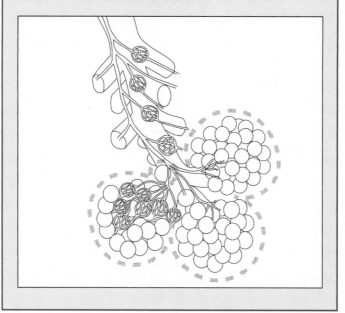

A close look at hyperinflated alveoli

In a hyperinflated lung, air becomes trapped in the alveoli, causing them to become hyperinflated as well.

Effect of PEEP on breath sounds

The use of positive end-expiratory pressure (PEEP) during mechanical ventilation increases functional residual capacity (the amount of air remaining in the airways at the end of normal expiration). Therefore, the lungs remain hyperinflated. Because increased amounts of air in the small airways and alveoli create a mismatch between the pleurae, chest wall, and the hyperinflated lung, breath sounds are diminished. **(38)**

No way out

Furthermore, the air trapped in a hyperinflated lung creates an impedance mismatch between the hyperinflated lung tissue, the pleurae, and chest wall. This condition further diminishes breath sounds. **(35)**

Conditions that cause hyperinflated lungs include chronic obstructive pulmonary disease (COPD), severe asthma, or the use of PEEP during mechanical ventilation. (See *Effect of PEEP on breath sounds*.)

Diminished by the process

In patients with COPD, the intensity of breath sounds directly relates to the severity of COPD. For example, patients with marked hyperinflation typically have increased anterior-to-posterior thoracic diameters and flattened and immobile diaphragms. The impedance mismatch caused by the trapped air and the decreased flow of air with each respiratory cycle, cause diminished breath sounds. Other signs and symptoms of COPD include a hyperresonant percussion note, dyspnea (a primary sign of severe COPD), and inaudible egophony, bronchophony, and whispered pectoriloquy.

When caring for a patient with COPD, monitor his breath sounds. If the sounds progress from diminished to absent, prepare for intubation and mechanical ventilation.

What you hear

In patients with COPD, you'll hear diminished or absent breath sounds throughout inspiration and expiration over the anterior, posterior, and lateral chest wall surfaces. **(36)** If breath sounds are audible, they sound soft with a low

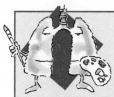

Inspired work

Auscultation sites in COPD

Due to a wide range of auscultatory findings, it's necessary to systematically auscultate the anterior chest wall, lateral chest wall, and posterior chest wall surfaces in patients with chronic obstructive pulmonary disease (COPD). Use these illustrations as guides when auscultating the lungs of a patient with COPD.

Anterior view

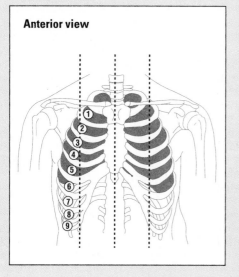

Posterior view

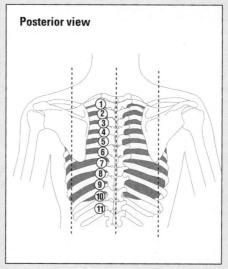

pitch. You can hear them best with the diaphragm of the stethoscope. (See *Auscultation sites in COPD*.)

Obesity

In an obese person, a thickened chest wall increases the distance between lung tissue and the chest wall surface, creating an impedance mismatch. This filters breath sounds as they're transmitted from the pleurae to the chest wall surface. **(37)**

What you hear

You'll hear diminished breath sounds over the anterior, posterior, and lateral chest wall surfaces. The location of fat pads determines where the breath sounds are most difficult to hear. For best results when auscultating an obese patient's lungs, ask him to sit up. Then ask him to take deep breaths through an open mouth while you listen.

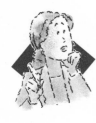

Quick quiz

1. When breath sounds are transmitted through a collection of air or fluid in the pleural space, sound transmission is:
  A. amplified.
  B. halted or filtered.
  C. unchanged.
  D. intermittently intensified.

Answer: B. When breath sounds are transmitted through a collection of air or fluid in the pleural space, sound transmission is halted or filtered.

2. During shallow breathing:
  A. less air flows through the airways during inspiration and expiration.
  B. turbulence in the airways increases.
  C. breath sounds become amplified.
  D. more air flows through the airways during inspiration and expiration.

Answer: A. During shallow breathing, less air flows through the airways during inspiration and expiration. Turbulence decreases, and breath sounds are diminished.

3. If a mainstem bronchus becomes obstructed:
  A. breath sounds are absent in the lower lobe.
  B. breath sounds are absent proximal to the obstruction.
  C. breath sounds are diminished proximal to the obstruction.
  D. breath sounds are absent throughout the entire affected lung.

Answer: D. If a mainstem bronchus becomes obstructed, breath sounds are absent throughout the entire affected lung.

4. Pneumothorax is:
    A. an accumulation of air in the mediastinum.
    B. an accumulation of air in the normally airless pleural space.
    C. immediately identifiable on auscultation.
    D. recognized by the absence of breath sounds.

Answer: B. Pneumothorax is an accumulation of air in the normally airless pleural space. A small pneumothorax may not alter breath sound intensity enough to be heard during auscultation. However, diminished or absent breath sounds usually accompany pneumothorax.

5. When a patient with COPD progresses from diminished to absent breath sounds:
    A. obtain nasal oxygen and a cannula.
    B. monitor vital sign every 4 hours.
    C. prepare for intubation and mechanical ventilation.
    D. suction the patient to clear the airway.

Answer: C. When a patient with COPD progresses from diminished to absent breath sounds, prepare for intubation and mechanical ventilation.

6. During inspiration, contractions of the dome-shaped diaphragm:
    A. expand the upper rib cage.
    B. force the abdominal contents upward and out.
    C. decrease the length of the lungs.
    D. lower intrapulmonary pressure.

Answer: D. During inspiration, the dome-shaped diaphragm contracts, which expands the lower rib cage and forces the abdominal contents downward and out, thereby increasing the length of the lungs. This process lowers intrapulmonary pressure and allows air to flow into the airways.

Scoring

☆☆☆ If you answered all six questions correctly, fabulous! You should feel inflated by your success over diminished breath sounds.

☆☆ If you answered four or five questions correctly, wonderful! There's no absence in your knowledge of breath sounds.

☆ If you answered fewer than four questions correctly, don't feel diminished. Learning about breath sounds, just like breathing itself, is simply a matter of repetition.

Adventitious sounds: Crackles

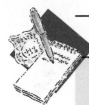

Just the facts

In this chapter, you'll learn:

♦ causes of crackles

♦ characteristics of late inspiratory crackles

♦ characteristics of early inspiratory and expiratory crackles.

Adventitious sounds at a glance

Over the years, terms used to classify adventitious breath sounds have changed repeatedly. Attempts have been made to make the terms clearer or more esthetic, or to characterize the sounds according to acoustic quality or musical tone. Unfortunately, these changes have often resulted in confusion.

Timing isn't everything

Currently, adventitious sounds are classified according to their acoustic quality, timing, and frequency waveforms. These sounds are further described as being discontinuous or continuous. Continuous sounds include wheezes (previously called *sibilant rales* or *sibilant rhonchi*) and low-pitched wheezes (previously called *sonorous rales* or *sonorous rhonchi*). Remember that the term *rhonchi* is still commonly used in the clinical setting, rather than *low-pitched wheezes*. These sounds are discussed in detail in the next chapter.

Putting a fine point on it

Discontinuous sounds include fine crackles (previously called *fine rales* or *crepitations*) and coarse crackles

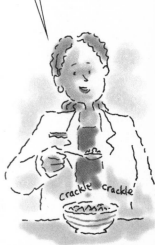

Crackles produce short, explosive or popping sounds that are described according to their pitch, timing, and location.

(previously called *rales* or *coarse rales*). **(39)** Keep in mind that fine crackles vary in intensity, so they may not always sound "fine." **(40)** In order for you to better understand these adventitious sounds, the discussion in this chapter categorizes crackles according to when you'll most likely hear them, such as during late inspiration or during early inspiration and expiration. Pleural crackles, which produce a unique sound, are also discussed.

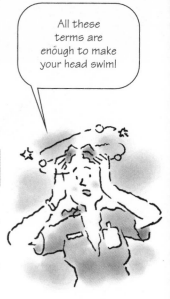

All these terms are enough to make your head swim!

Crackles at a glance

You'll hear crackles primarily through the chest wall with a stethoscope; however, you may also hear them at the patient's mouth, with or without a stethoscope. Described according to their pitch, timing, and location, crackles are short, explosive or popping sounds. The characteristics of these sounds change depending on the underlying cause. (See *Describing crackles*.)

It's generally known that crackles result when air bubbles through secretions in the airways; however, they can also be caused by a sudden, explosive opening of the airways.

Secretions as a cause

In such conditions as pulmonary edema and chronic bronchitis, the trachea and mainstem bronchi fill with sputum.

Describing crackles

When documenting the presence of crackles, you'll need to describe their timing, pitch, intensity, density, and duration:
• Timing refers to whether the sound occurs early, late, or in the middle of inspiration or expiration.
• Pitch refers to whether the sound has a high or low frequency.
• Intensity refers to whether the sound is loud or soft.
• Density refers to whether the crackles are profuse or scanty.
• Duration indicates the length of time that the crackles can be heard during inspiration or expiration.

Air bubbling through these secretions causes crackles to be heard on auscultation.

Because crackles occur mainly during inspiration, and because they may also occur in conditions in which sputum is absent, experts think another condition may cause crackles in the smaller airways.

> Air bubbling through secretions causes crackles to be heard on auscultation.

Opening airways as a cause

Normally, the peripheral airways in the lung bases close at the end of expiration. Those airways remain closed as inspiration begins, allowing air to flow first to the apex of each lung. The small airways distal to the closed peripheral airways remain underexpanded until airway pressures and external forces (such as those exerted with diaphragmatic movement and rib cage expansion) snap the airways open.

Grand opening

The sudden opening of multiple collapsed peripheral airways, along with the associated explosive changes in air pressures, likely produces crackles. This would help explain why crackles occur over the lung bases of a healthy person who inhales deeply following a maximum exhalation. This is probably also the cause of crackles heard in patients with atelectasis and interstitial lung disease.

Stuck in a routine

Crackles resulting from opening airways have a characteristic loudness and repetitive rhythm, which suggest that the airways open in the same sequence, at the same point in the respiratory cycle, and at the same approximate lung volumes.

You may hear crackles in the lung bases of elderly people and, occasionally, in other healthy individuals. These crackles clear with coughing and have no clinical significance.

> Just because you hear crackles doesn't mean I'm sick. Sometimes crackles occur because my peripheral airways suddenly reopen after a deep breath.

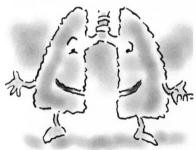

Conditions causing late inspiratory crackles

Late inspiratory crackles have a high-pitched, explosive sound of variable intensity and density. They're heard most commonly over dependent or poorly ventilated lung regions.

Conditions associated with these crackles include atelectasis, resolving lobar pneumonia, interstitial fibrosis, and left-sided heart failure.

Atelectasis

Atelectasis (the incomplete expansion of a lung area) may result from prolonged shallow breathing, gravitational forces that close airways and deflate the lung bases, and mucus plugging the airways. It typically occurs in postoperative and immobile patients as well as in those with impaired diaphragmatic function.

Use it or lose it

Atelectasis causes poor ventilation in the affected areas and may cause the segmental or lobar bronchi to collapse. If atelectasis occurs in the small peripheral airways, the patient may not have any symptoms. If, however, a larger airway is involved, the patient may have decreased chest wall movement, a dull percussion note, and bronchial breath sounds. You'll also hear egophony, bronchophony, and whispered pectoriloquy.

What you hear

The crackles associated with atelectasis result from the sudden opening of collapsed small airways and adjoining alveoli. These crackles are high-pitched, explosive sounds heard late in inspiration. **(43, 44)** Becoming more profuse toward the end of inspiration, they vary in intensity.

Fickle behavior

Because crackles associated with atelectasis are poorly transmitted to the chest wall surface, their intensity and density change with only a slight change

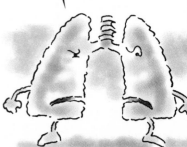

I knew I couldn't get away with not deep breathing. Those crackles give me away every time!

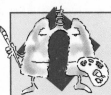

Inspired work

Auscultating for crackles in atelectasis

When assessing a postoperative patient who hasn't been coughing and deep breathing adequately, you may hear inspiratory crackles over the posterior bases of both lungs (shown below left). During your assessment, auscultate between the eighth and tenth intercostal spaces from the left posterior axillary line to the right posterior axillary line (shown below right).

Affected lung area

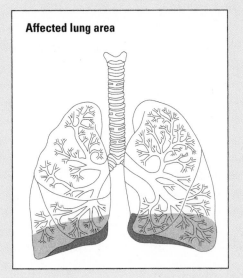

Posterior auscultatory sites

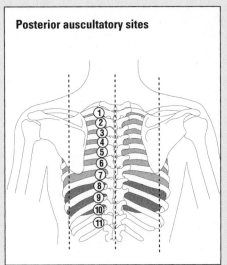

in stethoscope position. For example, you may hear profuse crackles in the dependent lung regions, but crackles may be scanty or absent in nondependent lung regions. You won't hear crackles at the patient's mouth. Crackles associated with atelectasis may also clear somewhat with coughing. (See *Auscultating for crackles in atelectasis.*)

The patient's ability to move or ambulate also affects these crackles. Prolonged immobility leads to ventilation of one area of the lung over another, causing atelectasis.

Lobar pneumonia

In patients with resolving lobar pneumonia, many alveoli are still filled with exudate while surrounding aveoli may have higher-than-normal aeration. A large increase in air pressure gradients occurs in the airways leading to the un-aerated alveoli.

Snapping to attention

As these airways snap open during late inspiration, crackles occur. These crackles sound similar to the late inspiratory crackles heard over areas with atelectasis; however, these crackles don't change if the patient coughs or changes position. **(45)**

What you hear

In a patient with right middle lobe pneumonia, you'll hear late inspiratory crackles over the right anterior chest wall surface between the third and fifth intercostal spaces. (See *Auscultating for crackles in lobar pneumonia.*)

Beginning late in inspiration, these crackles are typically high pitched and become more profuse toward the end of inspiration. **(46)**

Interstitial fibrosis

Diffuse interstitial fibrosis impairs or destroys alveoli by filling them with abnormal cells or by scarring the lung tissue. Unaffected alveoli are usually hyperaerated. The lungs become stiff, making inflation difficult, and airflow volumes usually decrease. A patient with a significant amount of lung involvement can have dyspnea and a cough.

Chronically late

During inspiration, the small airways most likely open late, causing the pressures in the diseased alveoli to fall more significantly than the pressures in the healthy alveoli. This leads to an increased pressure gradient, which generates repetitive late inspiratory crackles. **(47, 48)** Coughing doesn't affect the profusion of these crackles.

Heavy metal

Interstitial fibrosis may be caused by inhalation of heavy metals, the antibiotic nitrofurantoin, some chemothera-

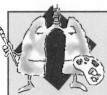

Inspired work

Auscultating for crackles in lobar pneumonia

In a patient with right middle lobe pneumonia, you'll hear late inspiratory crackles best over the right middle lobe (shown below left). Auscultate between the third and fifth intercostal spaces on the right anterior chest (shown below right).

Affected lung area

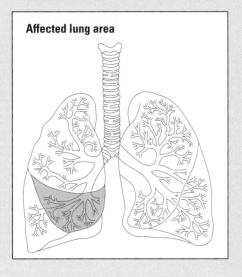

Anterior auscultatory sites

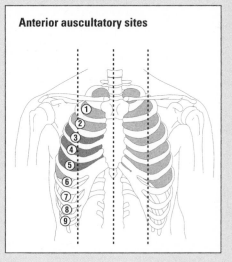

peutic agents, or prolonged inhalation of high concentrations of oxygen. It may also result from pulmonary sarcoidosis, rheumatoid arthritis, or scleroderma. In most cases, however, the etiology is unknown.

Crackles heard in a patient with known exposure to asbestos may be an early sign of asbestosis, a lung disease characterized by pulmonary inflammation and fibrosis. The longer the exposure to asbestos, the more profuse the crackles.

What you hear

In mild interstitial fibrosis, you'll typically hear crackles at the end of inspiration over dependent lung regions—usually over the lateral lung bases when the patient is sitting

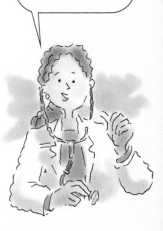

Whenever you auscultate crackles, be sure to ask the patient about exposure to asbestos. Crackles may be an early sign of the lung disease asbestosis.

Auscultating for crackles in interstitial fibrosis

In a patient with mild interstitial fibrosis, you'll usually hear late inspiratory crackles over the lateral lung bases at the end of inspiration. This illustration shows the areas to auscultate.

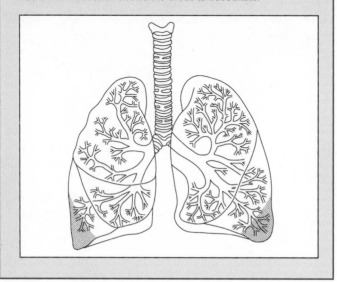

up. The crackles may disappear if the patient inhales deeply, holds his breath, or leans forward. However, they usually recur when he returns to an upright position. (See *Auscultating for crackles in interstitial fibrosis.*)

As interstitial fibrosis worsens, you'll hear crackles over both posterior lung bases as well as toward the apices. In later stages of the disease, you may hear crackles throughout inspiration that aren't affected by position changes.

Early on

In patients with interstitial fibrosis caused by early asbestosis, you'll hear crackles in the midaxillary area over the lateral lung bases. (See *Auscultating for crackles in early asbestosis.*)

Creeping crackles

As asbestosis progresses, you may hear crackles over the posterior bases as well as toward the apices. Heard during late inspiration, these crackles have a fine intensity and a

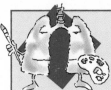

Inspired work

Auscultating for crackles in early asbestosis

When assessing a patient with early asbestosis, you'll most likely hear late inspiratory crackles over the lateral lung bases. Specifically, auscultate over the seventh and eighth intercostal spaces, as shown below.

Right lateral view

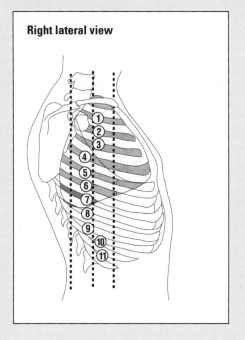

Left lateral view

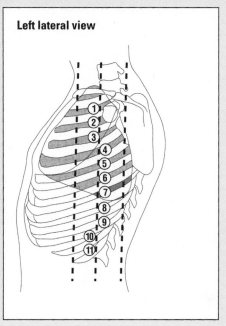

short, discontinuous duration. They have a high pitch that's heard best with the diaphragm of the stethoscope.

Left-sided heart failure

Left-sided heart failure leads to fluid accumulation in the lung tissue (pulmonary edema). This narrows the airways, causing them to open late during inspiration. The delayed opening forces the pressures to equalize rapidly, resulting in crackles. Common symptoms of left-sided heart failure include rapid, shallow breathing and mild hypoxia.

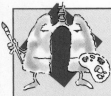

Inspired work

Auscultating for crackles in left-sided heart failure

With early left-sided heart failure and pulmonary edema, you'll hear fine, late inspiratory crackles over both posterior lung bases (shown below left). Focus your auscultation over the eighth, ninth, and tenth intercostal spaces (shown below right).

Affected lung area

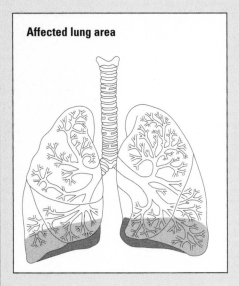

Posterior auscultatory sites

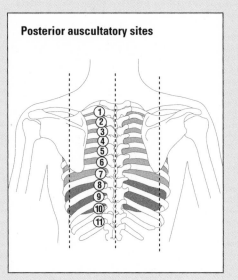

What you hear

In the early stages of left-sided heart failure and pulmonary edema, you'll hear profuse, high-pitched crackles over the posterior lung bases. **(49)** These crackles are inaudible at the mouth.

High tide

If pulmonary edema worsens, the airways become flooded with fluid, causing severe hypoxia. At this stage, you may hear low-pitched inspiratory and expiratory crackles at the mouth as well as over the entire chest wall surface. (See *Auscultating for crackles in left-sided heart failure.*)

Rattle trap

Later, as pulmonary edema worsens further, the crackles become loud, rattling, and profuse. You'll hear them throughout the chest during late inspiration, with the duration varying according to the degree of left-sided heart failure. The crackles have a low pitch that's heard best with either the bell or diaphragm of the stethoscope. **(50)**

Conditions causing early inspiratory and expiratory crackles

The crackles that occur during early inspiration and during expiration are also called *coarse crackles*. Heard over any chest wall area, the crackles are caused by diffuse airway obstruction. The sound most likely results when the large bronchi intermittently close and when a bolus of air flows past when the bronchi open.

Coarse behavior

Coarse crackles have a lower pitch than fine crackles. Although they're usually loud, coarse crackles may disappear after the patient coughs, but they're unaffected by the patient's position. Coarse crackles have an irregular rhythm that may be interrupted by short sequences of evenly spaced crackles with the same intensity. Coarse crackles often occur with chronic bronchitis and bronchiectasis.

Chronic bronchitis

Chronic exposure to airway irritants such as air pollution or, more commonly, cigarette smoke, triggers the proliferation and hypertrophy of mucous glands in the airways. This leads to excessive mucus production—as occurs in chronic bronchitis—which causes coarse crackles. Other clinical findings include cough, sputum production, and repeated respiratory infections. Chronic bronchitis can lead to chronic obstructive pulmonary disease. **(51)** (See *Lung findings in chronic bronchitis*, page 112.)

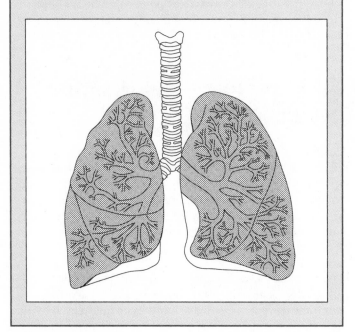

Lung findings in chronic bronchitis

This illustration shows the lung areas affected by chronic bronchitis. During auscultation, you'll hear early inspiratory crackles over the entire lung field.

What you hear

In patients with chronic bronchitis, you'll hear crackles early in inspiration over all chest wall surfaces and at the mouth. (See *Auscultating for crackles in chronic bronchitis.*)

The crackles will be scanty and low-pitched, and they won't be affected by the patient's position. **(52)**

Bronchiectasis

Bronchiectasis is the irreversible dilation of bronchi in selected lung segments. Fibrotic or atelectatic lung tissue surrounds the affected airways, which causes the airways to produce copious amounts of yellow or green sputum. A chest X-ray may reveal old inflammatory changes in the patient's lungs.

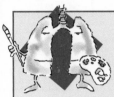

Inspired work

Auscultating for crackles in chronic bronchitis

Patients with chronic bronchitis typically have early inspiratory crackles. To hear these crackles, auscultate the areas highlighted in these illustrations.

Anterior view

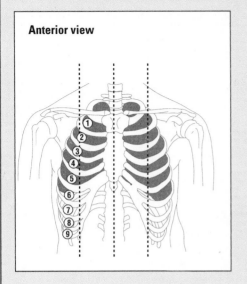

Posterior view

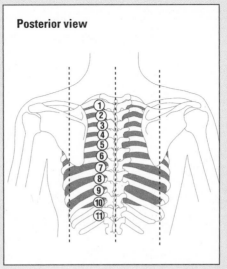

Causes of bronchiectasis include foreign body obstruction, tumor, viral or bacterial pneumonia (particularly multiple childhood pneumonias), chronic inflammatory or fibrotic lung disease, and tuberculosis. **(53)**

What you hear

In a patient with bronchiectasis in the left midlung and lower lung, you'll hear crackles over the anterior, posterior, and left lateral chest wall surfaces. (See *Auscultating for crackles in bronchiectasis*, page 114.)

The crackles are profuse, low-pitched, and coarser than those heard with chronic bronchitis. They occur during early or midinspiration. Although the crackles don't change with the patient's position, the number of crackles

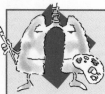

Inspired work

Auscultating for crackles in bronchiectasis

To auscultate the crackles associated with left midlung and lower lung bronchiectasis, listen over the anterior chest wall at the fourth, fifth, and sixth intercostal spaces. Then listen over the posterior chest wall at the seventh, eighth, ninth, and tenth intercostal spaces. These areas are highlighted in the illustrations below.

Anterior view

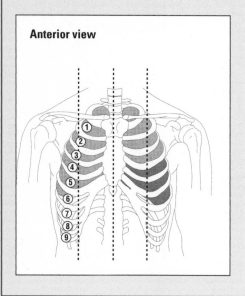

Posterior view

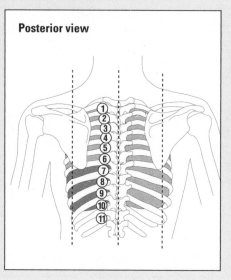

you hear may change if the patient coughs. **(54)** (See *Lung areas affected in bronchiectasis.*)

Conditions causing pleural crackles

If the visceral and parietal pleural surfaces become damaged by fibrin deposits or inflammatory or neoplastic cells, they lose their ability to glide silently over each other during breathing. Their movements become jerky and periodically delayed, producing loud, grating crackles known as *pleural crackles* or *pleural friction rub.* **(55, 56)**

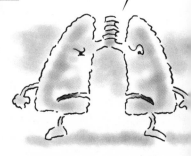

These pleurae are really starting to rub me the wrong way!

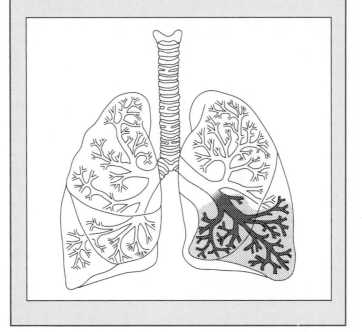

Lung areas affected in bronchiectasis

In a patient with bronchiectasis in the middle or lower left lung, you'll hear profuse early to midinspiratory crackles in the areas shown here.

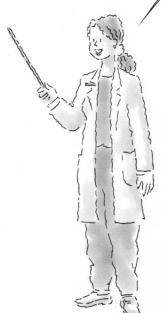

Pleural friction rub causes sharp pain during inspiration.

Silencing bad behavior

You may hear these crackles only during inspiration or during both inspiration and expiration. If fluid accumulates between the pleurae, the pleural crackles disappear.

Painful move

Patients with pleural friction rub usually complain of sharp pain during inspiration, causing them to splint the affected side to minimize muscle movement and chest expansion. Other findings include asymmetrical chest wall movement and rapid, shallow breathing.

Pleural crackles in the right midlung

This illustration shows a lung with damaged pleura in the right midlung. You'll hear the unique sounding pleural crackles over this area.

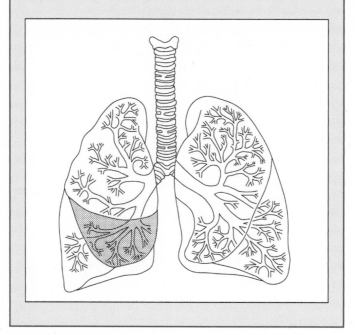

What you hear

In patients with pleural friction rub, you'll hear pleural crackles over the affected lung area. (See *Pleural crackles in the right midlung.*)

Pleural crackles over the middle of the right lung are loud and low-pitched and have a coarse, grating quality. **(55, 56)** Their duration is discontinuous. (See *Auscultating for crackles in pleural friction rub.*)

To distinguish between pleural friction rub and pericardial friction rub, ask the patient to hold his breath; if the rub continues, it's pericardial friction rub.

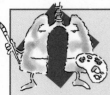

Inspired work

Auscultating for crackles in pleural friction rub

In a patient with a pleural friction rub in the right midlung, you'll hear pleural crackles over the fifth and sixth intercostal spaces between the right midclavicular and right midaxillary lines. These areas are highlighted in the illustrations below.

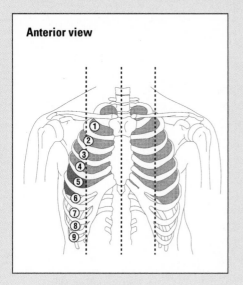

Anterior view

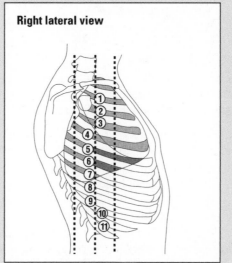

Right lateral view

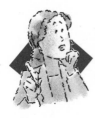

Quick quiz

1. Crackles produce a sound that's:
   A. high-pitched and tubular.
   B. loud and rumbling.
   C. short, explosive, or popping.
   D. long and sonorous.

Answer: C. Crackles produce short, explosive or popping sounds that are described according to their pitch, timing, and location.

2. Crackles in the smaller airways result from:
   A.   air bubbling through secretions.
   B.   shallow breathing.
   C.   sudden, explosive opening of airways.
   D.   vibration of the trachea and mainstem bronchus.

Answer: C. Crackles in the smaller airways result from the sudden, explosive opening of the airways.

3. Crackles that occur during early inspiration and during expiration are called:
   A.   coarse crackles.
   B.   fine crackles.
   C.   high-pitched crackles.
   D.   position-dependent crackles.

Answer: A. Coarse crackles occur during early inspiration and during expiration. They have a low pitch and may disappear with coughing but are unaffected by position.

4. In a postoperative patient who hasn't been coughing and deep breathing adequately, late inspiratory crackles are heard:
   A.   throughout the lungs.
   B.   in the trachea and mainstem bronchus.
   C.   over the right midlung.
   D.   over the posterior bases of both lungs.

Answer: D. In a postoperative patient who hasn't been coughing and deep breathing adequately, late inspiratory crackles are heard over the posterior bases of both lungs.

5. Pleural crackles are described as sounding:
   A.   soft and high-pitched.
   B.   loud, coarse, and grating.
   C.   low-pitched and musical.
   D.   loud, sonorous, and rumbling.

Answer: B. Pleural crackles are described as sounding loud, coarse, and grating.

Scoring

☆☆☆   If you answered all five questions correctly, stupendous! We're inspired by your knowledge of crackles.

☆☆   If you answered four questions correctly, way to go! You have a grasp of crackles that's sure to never expire.

☆   If you answered fewer than four questions correctly, don't feel deflated. It's never too late to become inspired by breath sounds.

Adventitious sounds: Wheezes

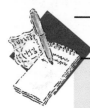

Just the facts

In this chapter, you'll learn:
♦ the origin of wheezes
♦ characteristics of expiratory polyphonic, fixed monophonic, sequential inspiratory, and random monophonic wheezes
♦ conditions associated with wheezes.

Wheezes at a glance

Wheezes are high-pitched, continuous breath sounds with frequencies of 200 Hz or greater and a duration of 250 milliseconds or more. Musical in tone, wheezes result when air passes through an extremely narrowed bronchus. The bronchus walls oscillate between being barely open to completely closed, which produces the audible sound of wheezes. (See *Airflow patterns and oscillations of a narrowed bronchus*, page 120.)

Conditions associated with wheezes include bronchospasm, airway thickening from mucosal swelling or muscle hypertrophy, inhalation of a foreign object, tumor, secretions, or dynamic airway compression.

Describing wheezes

When you detect wheezes during an auscultatory assessment, listen carefully to determine the timing, location, and pitch of these adventitious sounds. These characteristics, which may vary considerably, will reveal information about the patient's underlying condition.

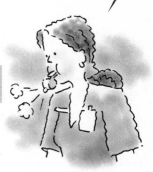

Just like the air passing through my whistle, air flowing through an extremely narrowed bronchus makes a musical sound.

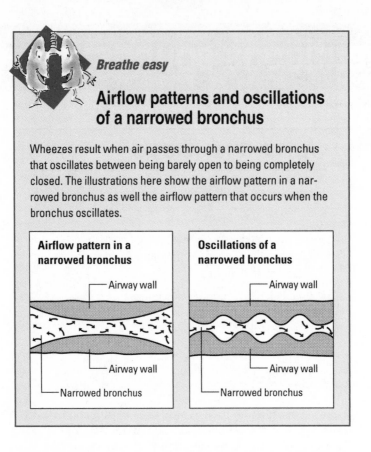

Breathe easy

Airflow patterns and oscillations of a narrowed bronchus

Wheezes result when air passes through a narrowed bronchus that oscillates between being barely open to being completely closed. The illustrations here show the airflow pattern in a narrowed bronchus as well the airflow pattern that occurs when the bronchus oscillates.

Airflow pattern in a narrowed bronchus

Airway wall

Airway wall

Narrowed bronchus

Oscillations of a narrowed bronchus

Airway wall

Airway wall

Narrowed bronchus

Timing

You'll describe your patient's wheezes according to their timing within the respiratory cycle.

It's about time!

You may hear wheezes during inspiration, expiration, or continuously throughout the respiratory cycle. Also, the patient's wheezes may be episodic (occurring only occasionally), or they may be chronic.

Location

Because lung tissue absorbs high-frequency sounds, you'll hear wheezes better when auscultating over the central airways. However, keep in mind that just because you auscultate a wheeze over the central airways doesn't mean that the sound originated there. The airways may simply be transmitting a sound produced in another part of the lung.

Mouthing off

Sometimes you'll hear wheezes at the patient's mouth. In fact, if the patient has a severe airway obstruction, you may hear wheezes at his mouth that you won't hear during auscultation of his chest wall. If you hear wheezes at the patient's mouth, and breath sounds are diminished or absent, be alert for impending respiratory failure.

Wheezes may be localized, occurring over isolated lung areas, or they may be diffuse, occurring throughout the lung field.

Pitch

The pitch, or frequency, of a wheeze can vary widely over a five-octave range. These differences in pitch result from variations in the size and elasticity of the airway as well as the airflow through the narrowed bronchus. Theoretically, large, flabby airways generate low-pitched sounds when narrowed; smaller, stiff airways generate high-pitched sounds when narrowed.

Don't everyone talk at once!

Wheezes having different pitches may occur at the same time, or they may overlap. Also, the pitch of a single wheeze may change during inspiration and expiration. During auscultation, you may hear wheezes that produce a single musical note, which may vary in duration and may overlap. These are called *monophonic wheezes*. Other wheezes, which produce multiple musical tones simultaneously, are called *polyphonic wheezes*.

Understanding types of wheezes

The main categories of wheezes include expiratory polyphonic wheezes, fixed monophonic wheezes, sequential inspiratory wheezes, and random monophonic wheezes. Stridor is another type of wheeze, which we'll also discuss.

Memory jogger

To help you remember which characteristics to assess when listening to a patient's wheezes, imagine you're a batter stepping up to the plate:

- Watch your **timing** when taking a swing.

- Know the **location** of incoming balls.

- Wait for the perfect **pitch.**

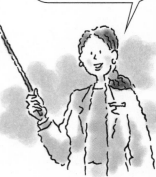

Remember that "mono" means "one." Therefore, monophonic wheezes produce only one tone. "Poly" means "many," so polyphonic wheezes produce multiple tones.

Expiratory polyphonic wheezes

Polyphonic wheezes, which produce several unrelated musical sounds, most likely result from the dynamic compression of the large airways during expiration. Because lung compliance and airway resistance don't vary between lung regions, you'll hear these wheezes throughout the lung field. (See *Expiratory polyphonic wheezes*.)

An embargo on airflow

If you auscultate polyphonic wheezes in a patient who isn't in respiratory distress, suspect a condition causing widespread airflow obstruction, such as chronic asthma or chronic bronchitis. These conditions alter peripheral airway resistance, airway mechanics, and the lung's elastic recoil properties throughout both lungs. In turn, this affects the timing of dynamic airway compression of the large airways, which alters the patient's breath sounds.

Domino effect

For example, if a patient with asthma exhales forcefully several times, the central bronchi compress first when elastic recoil of the airways is low or when peripheral airway resistance is high. This compression produces a series of sounds, beginning with a monophonic wheeze and

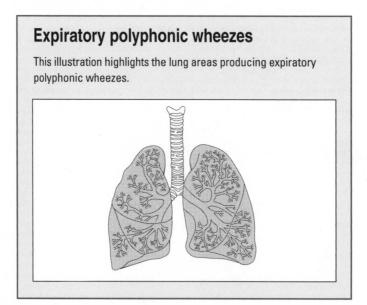

Expiratory polyphonic wheezes

This illustration highlights the lung areas producing expiratory polyphonic wheezes.

quickly followed by bitonal sounds. Very soon, the full complement of sounds that make up polyphonic wheezes are audible through the stethoscope.

You may occasionally hear expiratory polyphonic wheezes in a healthy person during a forced expiration. In this instance, the wheezes result when maximal forced expiration triggers simultaneous dynamic compression of all the airways.

What you hear

To hear expiratory polyphonic wheezes, listen with the diaphragm of the stethoscope over the anterior, posterior, and lateral chest wall surfaces as the patient exhales. (See *Auscultating for expiratory polyphonic wheezes.*)

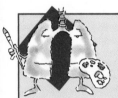

Inspired work

Auscultating for expiratory polyphonic wheezes

When auscultating expiratory polyphonic wheezes, have the patient exhale while you listen over his anterior, posterior, and lateral chest wall surfaces.

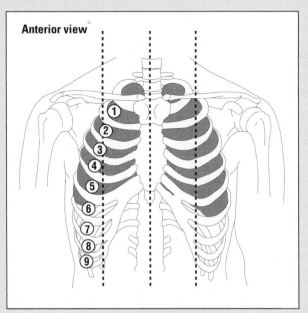

Anterior view

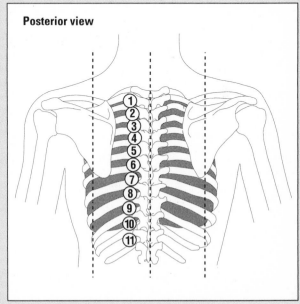

Posterior view

Loud and widely transmitted, these multiple musical tones begin simultaneously and have a continuous duration. They have a high pitch that remains constant and then rises sharply at the end of expiration. **(57, 58)**

Fixed monophonic wheezes

Fixed monophonic wheezes produce a single musical tone of a constant pitch. These wheezes result when air flows rapidly through a large, partially obstructed bronchus. Such an obstruction may result from a tumor, a foreign body, bronchial stenosis, or an intrabronchial granuloma.

Don't be so rigid

If the patient has bronchial stenosis, the pitch of inspiratory and expiratory monophonic wheezes will vary, depending on the rigidity of the airway. Monophonic wheezes may disappear when the patient lies on his back or turns from side to side. (See *Fixed monophonic wheezes*.)

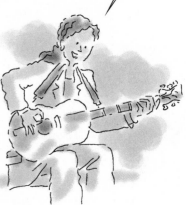

When you listen for fixed monophonic wheezes, you'll hear a single musical tone of a constant pitch.

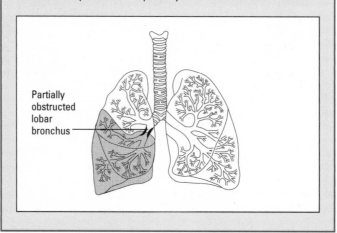

Fixed monophonic wheezes

This illustration highlights the lung areas producing monophonic wheezes in a patient with a partially obstructed lobar bronchus.

Partially obstructed lobar bronchus

What you hear

Transmitted throughout the lungs, fixed monophonic wheezes have a low pitch heard best with the diaphragm of the stethoscope. **(59, 60)** If the patient has a partially obstructed right lobar bronchus, you'll hear fixed monophonic wheezes over the anterior, posterior, and right lateral chest wall surfaces. (See *Auscultating for fixed monophonic wheezes.*)

Fixed monophonic wheezes are usually loud, and their duration is continuous. You may hear them during inspiration, expiration, or throughout the respiratory cycle.

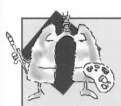

Inspired work

Auscultating for fixed monophonic wheezes

To hear fixed monophonic wheezes in a patient with a partially obstructed right lobar bronchus, focus your auscultation over the third, fourth, fifth, and sixth intercostal spaces anteriorly and the fifth, sixth, seventh, eighth, ninth, and tenth intercostal spaces posteriorly. These areas are highlighted in the illustrations below.

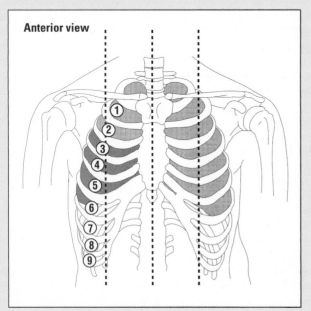

Anterior view

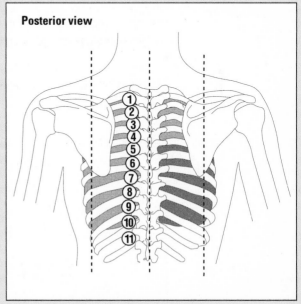

Posterior view

Sequential inspiratory wheezes

Sequential inspiratory wheezes, which produce a single musical tone, result when airways in unaerated lung regions open late during inspiration. The rapid inflow of air causes the airway walls to vibrate, generating a series of inspiratory wheezes.

You'll occasionally hear sequential inspiratory wheezes over the lung bases of patients with interstitial fibrosis, asbestosis, or fibrosing alveolitis. In patients with interstitial fibrosis, you may hear a single, short inspiratory wheeze — or a brief sequence of monophonic inspiratory wheezes with different pitches — along with the crackles usually associated with this disorder. **(61, 62)** (See *Sequential inspiratory wheezes.*)

What you hear

You'll usually hear sequential inspiratory wheezes over the lateral and posterior lung bases. (See *Auscultating for sequential inspiratory wheezes.*)

Sequential inspiratory wheezes have a loud intensity and a high pitch heard best with the diaphragm of the stethoscope. Continuous in duration, you'll hear them

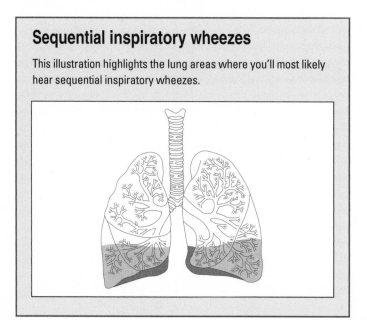

Sequential inspiratory wheezes

This illustration highlights the lung areas where you'll most likely hear sequential inspiratory wheezes.

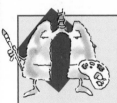

Inspired work

Auscultating for sequential inspiratory wheezes

To hear sequential inspiratory wheezes, auscultate over the posterior chest wall surface at the eighth, ninth, and tenth intercostal spaces (shown below left) and over the lateral chest wall surface at the seventh and eighth intercostal spaces (shown below center and right).

Posterior view

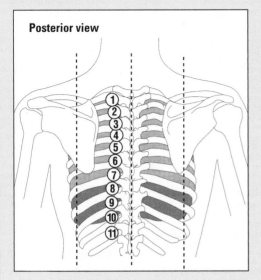

Right lateral view

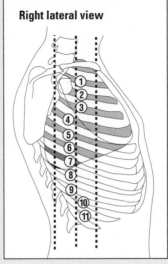

Left lateral view

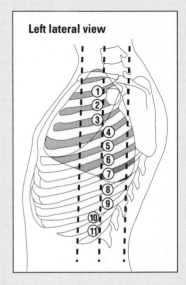

throughout inspiration, but they're more predominant in late inspiration. **(61, 62)**

Random monophonic wheezes

When bronchospasm or mucosal swelling narrows the airways, single or multiple monophonic wheezes may occur during inspiration, expiration, or throughout the respiratory cycle. Multiple wheezes may occur randomly and vary in duration. (See *Random monophonic wheezes*, page 128.)

Loud mouth

The intensity of the wheeze will vary, depending on the area producing the sound. For example, random monophonic wheezes produced in the large central airways are

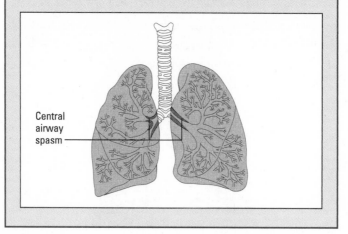

Random monophonic wheezes

This illustration highlights the areas where you'll hear random monophonic wheezes in a patient with central airway spasm.

Central
airway
spasm

loud and widely transmitted throughout the lung. In fact, you'll hear them at the patient's mouth while standing a distance away. **(63, 64)**

The silent type

In contrast, random monophonic wheezes produced in the peripheral airways are weaker. Because the sounds are filtered as they travel to the chest wall, you'll hear them only when auscultating over the chest wall.

Shifting alliances

Random monophonic wheezes typically occur in patients with severe status asthmaticus. In status asthmaticus, airway resistance increases. At the same time, dynamic airway compression shifts from the central airways toward the smaller peripheral airways, where the airflow rate is too low to produce airway wall vibrations or sounds.

Status asthmaticus triggers progressive airway obstruction, producing a predictable pattern of wheezing. Initially audible only during expiration, monophonic wheezes eventually occur throughout the respiratory cycle. Because these high-frequency sounds travel through larger airways, you'll also hear them at the patient's mouth.

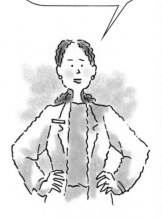

If you're caring for an asthmatic patient and his wheezes suddenly disappear, get help immediately! His condition could be life-threatening.

It's a trap!

As status asthmaticus becomes more severe, air trapping and severe airway narrowing occurs, which forces the site of dynamic airway compression to move toward the lung periphery. As a result, all wheezes heard over the chest wall disappear. Called *silent chest*, this phenomenon is commonly accompanied by hypercapnia (increased carbon dioxide levels in the blood) and acidosis, both of which are life-threatening.

What you hear

You'll usually hear random monophonic wheezes over the anterior, posterior, and lateral chest wall surfaces. (See *Auscultating for random monophonic wheezes*.)

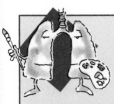

Inspired work

Auscultating for random monophonic wheezes

When monitoring a patient for random monophonic wheezes, auscultate the patient's anterior, posterior, and lateral chest wall surfaces. These areas are highlighted in the illustrations below.

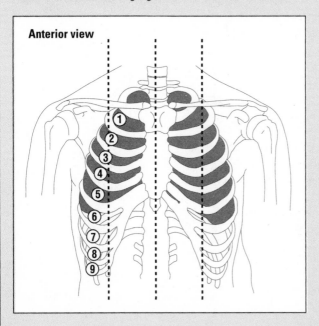

Anterior view

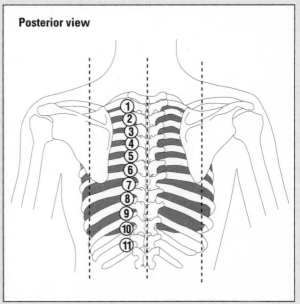

Posterior view

Typically loud with a continuous duration, these wheezes have a high pitch heard best with the diaphragm of the stethoscope. They occur throughout the respiratory cycle. Patients with random monophonic wheezes typically have a prolonged expiration.

Stridor

When laryngeal spasm and mucosal swelling contract the vocal cords and narrow the airway, stridor results.

Hard to miss

A very loud musical sound, stridor can usually be heard without a stethoscope while at a distance from the patient. The monophonic wheeze of stridor typically occurs during inspiration, however, as airway constriction increases, it may become audible throughout the respiratory cycle. Its intensity distinguishes it from other monophonic wheezes. **(73)**

Stridor usually occurs with severe upper respiratory infections. It may also occur with whooping cough, laryngeal tumors, tracheal stenosis, and aspiration of a foreign object.

What you hear

When severe, stridor is audible without a stethoscope. If the patient has a less-pronounced laryngeal spasm, auscultate over the larynx to hear the sound. Very loud with a continuous duration, stridor usually occurs during inspiration but may also occur throughout the respiratory cycle. Its high pitch resembles a crowing sound. **(65, 66)**

If the patient with stridor is drooling, realize that the epiglottis may be severely swollen. Because any stimulus may worsen the airway occlusion, avoid examining the patient's mouth. Initiate emergency measures and prepare for intubation. If the edema is severe enough to prohibit intubation, prepare for an emergency tracheotomy.

Use extreme caution if you notice that a patient with stridor is drooling. Any stimulus could trigger a complete airway occlusion.

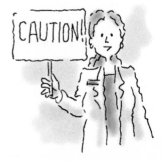

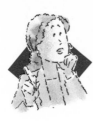

Quick quiz

1. Wheezes are:
A. rumbling sounds.
B. grating sounds.
C. inaudible sounds.
D. musical sounds.

Answer: D. Wheezes are musical sounds generated when air passes through a bronchus so narrowed that it's almost closed.

2. Be alert for impending respiratory failure if your patient has wheezes that are audible at the mouth along with:
A. fine crackles.
B. bronchial breath sounds.
C. diminished or absent breath sounds.
D. mostly vesicular breath sounds.

Answer: C. Be alert for impending respiratory failure if your patient has wheezes that are audible at the mouth along with diminished or absent breath sounds.

3. Fixed monophonic wheezes result from:
A. the oscillations of a large, partially obstructed bronchus.
B. a collection of fluid in the pleura.
C. airways that open late in inspiration in unaerated lung regions.
D. dynamic compression of large airways during expiration.

Answer: A. Fixed, monophonic wheezes result from the oscillations of a large, partially obstructed bronchus.

4. Random, monophonic wheezes occur in patients who have:
A. pulmonary edema.
B. pulmonary fibrosis.
C. status asthmaticus.
D. a pleural friction rub.

Answer: C. Random, monophonic wheezes occur in patients who have status asthmaticus.

5.   Stridor results from:
  A.   obstructed bronchi.
  B.   laryngeal spasm and mucosal swelling.
  C.   compression of the large airways during expiration.
  D.   narrowed bronchi.

Answer: B. Stridor results from laryngeal spasm and mucosal swelling.

Scoring

☆☆☆   If you answered all five questions correctly, incredible! You've breezed through this chapter on wheezes.

☆☆   If you answered four questions correctly, excellent work! You can now make a pitch for being a master of these high-frequency breath sounds.

☆   If you answered fewer than four questions correctly, don't despair. It might be "adventitious" to read this chapter again.

Respiratory disorders

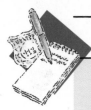

Just the facts

In this chapter, you'll learn:

♦ causes and pathophysiology of common respiratory disorders

♦ signs and symptoms of common respiratory disorders

♦ treatment and nursing care for common respiratory disorders.

Common respiratory disorders at a glance

Auscultation skills discussed in the previous chapters are important tools you'll use when caring for patients with respiratory disorders. The respiratory disorders introduced earlier are complex, and you need to know what to look for, how each disorder is treated, and what to do for the patient.

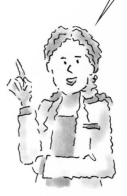

Gaining an understanding of common respiratory disorders will help you apply your auscultation skills more effectively.

Acute respiratory distress syndrome

A form of pulmonary edema that leads to acute respiratory failure, acute respiratory distress syndrome (ARDS) results from increased permeability of the alveolocapillary membrane. Although severe ARDS may be fatal, recovering patients may have little or no permanent lung damage.

What causes it

ARDS may result from:
• aspiration of gastric contents
• sepsis (primarily gram-negative)

• trauma (such as lung contusion, head injury, and long-bone fracture with fat emboli)
• oxygen toxicity
• viral, bacterial, or fungal pneumonia
• microemboli (fat or air emboli or disseminated intravascular coagulation)
• drug overdose (such as barbiturates, glutethimide, and opioids)
• blood transfusion
• smoke or chemical inhalation (such as nitrous oxide, chlorine, ammonia, and organophosphates)
• hydrocarbon or paraquat ingestion
• pancreatitis, uremia, or, in rare cases, miliary tuberculosis (TB)
• near drowning.

Pathophysiology

In ARDS, fluid accumulates in the lung interstitium, alveolar spaces, and small airways, causing the lung to stiffen. This impairs ventilation and reduces oxygenation of pulmonary capillary blood. (See *What happens in ARDS.*)

What to look for

Assess your patient for the following signs and symptoms:
• rapid, shallow breathing; dyspnea; and hypoxemia
• intercostal and suprasternal retractions, crackles, and rhonchi
• tachycardia
• restlessness, apprehension, mental sluggishness, and motor dysfunction.

What tests tell you

• Arterial blood gas (ABG) values on room air show a partial pressure of arterial oxygen (Pao_2) below 60 mm Hg and partial pressure of arterial carbon dioxide ($Paco_2$) below 35 mm Hg. As ARDS becomes more severe, ABG values show respiratory acidosis, with $Paco_2$ values elevated above 45 mm Hg. Metabolic acidosis is also present, with bicarbonate (HCO_3^-) values below 22 mEq/L. The patient's Pao_2 decreases despite oxygen therapy.
• Pulmonary artery (PA) catheterization helps identify the cause of pulmonary edema by evaluating pulmonary artery wedge pressure; allows collection of pulmonary

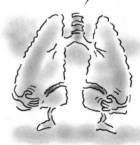

Ow! All this fluid in my interstitium has made me feel so stiff.

Breathe easy

What happens in ARDS

The illustrations below show the development of acute respiratory distress syndrome (ARDS).

Injury reduces normal blood flow to the lungs, allowing platelets to aggregate. These platelets release substances, such as serotonin (S), bradykinin (B), and histamine (H), that inflame and damage the alveolar membrane and later increase capillary permeability.

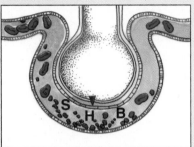

Histamines (H) and other inflammatory substances increase capillary permeability. Fluids shift into the interstitial space.

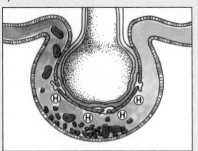

As capillary permeability increases, proteins and more fluid leak out, causing pulmonary edema.

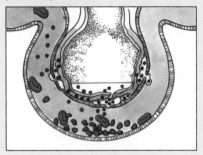

Fluid in the alveoli and decreased blood flow damage surfactant in the alveoli. This reduces the alveolar cells' ability to produce more surfactant. Without surfactant, alveoli collapse, impairing gas exchange.

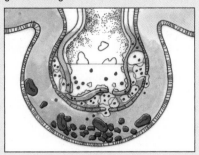

The patient breathes faster, but sufficient oxygen (O_2) can't cross the alveolar capillary membrane. Carbon dioxide (CO_2), however, crosses more easily and is lost with every exhalation. Both O_2 and CO_2 levels in the blood decrease.

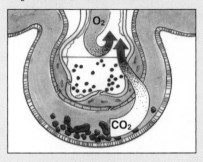

Pulmonary edema worsens. Meanwhile, inflammation leads to fibrosis, which further impedes gas exchange. The resulting hypoxemia leads to respiratory acidosis.

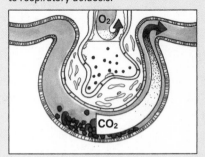

artery blood, which shows decreased oxygen saturation (Sao_2) (a sign of tissue hypoxia); measures pulmonary artery pressure; and measures cardiac output by thermodilution techniques.

• Serial chest X-rays initially show bilateral infiltrates. In later stages, the X-rays have a ground-glass appearance and, as hypoxemia becomes irreversible, "whiteouts" are seen in both lung fields.
• Other tests may be performed to detect infections, drug ingestion, or pancreatitis.

How it's treated

Treatment aims to correct the underlying cause of ARDS before it leads to potentially fatal complications.

Air pump

Supportive medical care includes humidified oxygen through a tight-fitting mask, allowing the use of continuous positive airway pressure. When hypoxemia doesn't respond to these measures, patients require ventilatory support with intubation, volume ventilation, and positive end-expiratory pressure. Other supportive measures include fluid restriction, diuretics, and correction of electrolyte and acid-base abnormalities.

Relax and take a deep breath...

Patients who receive mechanical ventilation commonly require sedatives and opioids or neuromuscular blocking agents, such as vecuronium and pancuronium, to minimize anxiety. Decreasing anxiety enhances ventilation by reducing oxygen consumption and carbon dioxide production.

If given early, a short course of high-dose steroids may be beneficial to patients with ARDS that results from fat emboli or chemical injury to the lungs. Treatment with sodium bicarbonate may be necessary to reverse severe metabolic acidosis. Fluids and vasopressors are administered to maintain the patient's blood pressure. Nonviral infections require antimicrobial drugs.

What to do

ARDS requires careful monitoring and supportive care. To prepare your patient for transfer to an intensive care unit (ICU), follow these steps:
• Frequently assess the patient's respiratory status. Be alert for retractions on inspiration. Note the rate, rhythm, and depth of respirations and watch for dyspnea and the use of accessory muscles of respiration. On auscultation,

listen for adventitious or diminished breath sounds. Check for pink, frothy sputum, which may indicate pulmonary edema.
• Observe and document the hypoxemic patient's neurologic status. Assess his level of consciousness (LOC) and observe for mental sluggishness.
• Maintain a patent airway by suctioning the patient as needed.
• Closely monitor heart rate and rhythm and blood pressure.
• Reposition the patient often and observe for hypotension, increased secretions, or elevated body temperature—all signs of deterioration.
• Evaluate the patient. After successful treatment, he should have normal ABG values; a normal respiratory rate, depth, and pattern; and clear breath sounds. (See *Teaching the patient with ARDS*.)

> ### Teaching the patient with ARDS
>
> Advise the patient with acute respiratory distress syndrome (ARDS) that recovery will take some time and that strength will return gradually. Provide emotional support as needed. Also, if the patient requires mechanical ventilation, provide him with an alternate means of communication.

Acute respiratory failure

Acute respiratory failure (ARF) occurs when the lungs no longer meet the body's metabolic needs.

A 50-50 proposition

In patients with essentially normal lung tissue, a $Paco_2$ above 50 mm Hg and a Pao_2 below 50 mm Hg usually indicate ARF. These limits, however, don't apply to patients with chronic obstructive pulmonary disease (COPD), who commonly have a consistently high $Paco_2$ and low Pao_2. In patients with COPD, only acute deterioration in ABG values, with corresponding clinical deterioration, indicates ARF.

What causes it

ARF may develop from any condition that increases the work of breathing and decreases the respiratory drive, including:
• respiratory tract infections (such as bronchitis and pneumonia—the most common precipitating factors)
• bronchospasm
• accumulated secretions due to cough suppression
• central nervous system (CNS) depression from head trauma or injudicious use of sedatives, opioids, tranquilizers, or oxygen

- cardiovascular disorders (such as myocardial infarction [MI], heart failure, or pulmonary emboli)
- airway irritants (such as smoke or fumes)
- endocrine and metabolic disorders (such as myxedema or metabolic alkalosis)
- thoracic abnormalities (including chest trauma, pneumothorax, or thoracic or abdominal surgery).

Pathophysiology

ARF results from impaired gas exchange, when the lungs don't oxygenate the blood adequately and fail to prevent carbon dioxide retention.

Falling down on the job

Any condition associated with hypoventilation (a reduction in the volume of air moving into and out of the lung), ventilation-perfusion ($\dot{V}/\dot{Q}$) mismatch (too little ventilation with normal blood flow or too little blood flow with normal ventilation), or intrapulmonary shunting (right-to-left shunting in which blood passes from the heart's right side to its left without being oxygenated) can cause ARF if left untreated.

What to look for

Patients with ARF experience hypoxemia and acidemia affecting all body organs, especially the central nervous, respiratory, and cardiovascular systems. Although specific symptoms vary with the underlying cause, you should always assess for:
- altered respirations (increased, decreased, or normal rate; shallow, deep, or alternating shallow and deep respirations; possible cyanosis; crackles, rhonchi, wheezes, or diminished breath sounds on chest auscultation)
- cardiac arrhythmias (from myocardial hypoxia)
- tachycardia (occurs early in response to low PaO_2)
- pulmonary hypertension (increased pressures on the right side of the heart, elevated neck veins, enlarged liver, and peripheral edema)
- altered mentation (restlessness, confusion, loss of concentration, irritability, tremulousness, diminished tendon reflexes, or papilledema).

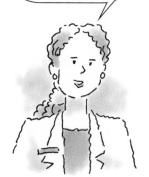

Be alert for any condition causing impaired gas exchange. Left untreated, ARF may result.

What tests tell you

• Progressive deterioration in ABG levels and pH, when compared with the patient's baseline values, strongly suggests ARF. (In patients with essentially normal lung tissue, a pH value below 7.35 usually indicates ARF. However, COPD patients display an even greater deviation in pH values, along with deviations in $Paco_2$ and Pao_2.)
• Serum HCO_3^- shows increased levels, either because of metabolic alkalosis or from metabolic compensation for chronic respiratory acidosis.
• Complete blood count (CBC) reveals low hematocrit and hemoglobin levels (possibly from blood loss), indicating decreased oxygen-carrying capacity. CBC will also show an elevated white blood cell (WBC) count if ARF results from bacterial infection (pathogens identified using Gram stain and sputum culture).
• Serum electrolyte levels reveal hypokalemia, possibly from compensatory hyperventilation (an attempt to correct alkalosis), and hypochloremia, which is common in metabolic alkalosis.
• Chest X-rays show pulmonary abnormalities, such as emphysema, atelectasis, lesions, pneumothorax, infiltrates, and effusions.
• Electrocardiogram (ECG) discloses arrhythmias, which commonly suggest cor pulmonale and myocardial hypoxia.

How it's treated

In COPD patients, ARF is an emergency requiring cautious oxygen therapy (using nasal prongs or a Venturi mask) to raise the patient's Pao_2.

Bringing in the heavy equipment

If significant respiratory acidosis persists, mechanical ventilation through an endotracheal (ET) or a tracheostomy tube may be necessary. High-frequency ventilation may be used if the patient doesn't respond to conventional mechanical ventilation. Prone positioning may also prove beneficial. Treatment routinely includes antibiotics for infection, bronchodilators and, possibly, steroids.

What to do

ARF requires close attention to airway patency and oxygen supply. Follow these steps:
• To reverse hypoxemia, administer oxygen at appropriate concentrations to maintain Pao_2 at a minimum of 50 mm Hg. Patients with COPD usually require only small amounts of supplemental oxygen. Watch for a positive response, such as improvement in ABG results and the patient's breathing and color.
• Maintain a patent airway. If the patient is intubated and lethargic, turn him every 1 to 2 hours. Use postural drainage and chest physiotherapy to help clear secretions.
• In an intubated patient, suction the airways before and after hyperoxygenation, as required. Assess for changes in quantity, consistency, and color of sputum. To prevent aspiration and reduce the risk of ventilator-associated pneumonia, always suction the oropharynx and the area above the cuff of the ET tube before deflating the cuff. Provide humidity to liquefy secretions.
• Observe the patient closely for respiratory arrest. Auscultate for breath sounds. Monitor ABG levels and report changes immediately.

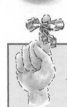

> When giving oxygen to a patient with COPD, start with a low flow rate; usually, that's all that will be necessary.

Checks and balances

• Monitor serum electrolyte levels and correct imbalances; monitor fluid balance by recording fluid intake and output and daily weight.
• Check the cardiac monitor for arrhythmias.
• If the patient requires mechanical ventilation and is unstable, he'll probably be transferred to an ICU. Arrange for his safe transfer.
• If the patient isn't on mechanical ventilation and is retaining carbon dioxide, encourage him to cough and breathe deeply with pursed lips. If the patient is alert, teach and encourage him to use an incentive spirometer.
• Evaluate the patient. Make sure that ABG values are normal, with a Pao_2 greater than 50 mm Hg, and that the patient can make a normal respiratory effort.

Memory jogger

When caring for a patient receiving oxygen through an endotracheal (ET) tube, remember to keep the acronym **SAPH** in mind:

Suction before and after hyperoxygenation as required.

Assess sputum for changes in quantity, consistency, and color.

Prevent aspiration by suctioning the oropharynx and area above the ET tube before deflating the cuff.

Humidify to liquefy secretions.

Asbestosis

Asbestosis is characterized by diffuse interstitial pulmonary fibrosis. Prolonged exposure to airborne asbestos particles causes pleural plaques and tumors of the pleura and peritoneum. Asbestosis may develop 15 to 20 years after the period of regular exposure to asbestos has ended. (See *A close look at asbestosis.*)

Hazardous duty

People at high risk for asbestosis include workers in the mining, milling, construction, fireproofing, and textile industries. Asbestos is also used in paints, plastics, and brake and clutch linings. Cigarette smoking increases the risk of asbestosis. In fact, an asbestos worker who smokes is 90 times more likely to develop lung cancer than a smoker who has never worked with asbestos.

Family matters

Family members of asbestos workers may develop asbestosis from exposure to stray fibers shaken off the workers' clothing. The general public may be exposed to

A close look at asbestosis

After years of exposure to asbestos, healthy lung tissue progresses to massive pulmonary fibrosis, as shown below.

Healthy lung tissue

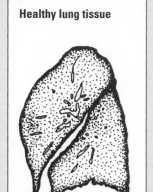

Simple asbestosis

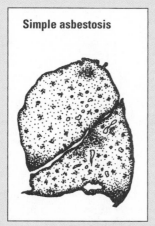

Progressive massive fibrosis

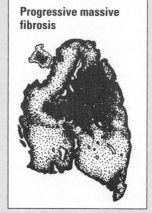

fibrous asbestos dust in deteriorating buildings or in waste piles from asbestos plants.

What causes it

Asbestosis results from prolonged inhalation of asbestos fibers.

Pathophysiology

Asbestosis begins when inhaled asbestos fibers travel down the airway and penetrate respiratory bronchioles and alveolar walls.

Going undercover

The fibers become encased in a brown, iron-rich, protein-like sheath in sputum or lung tissue. Interstitial fibrosis may develop in lower lung zones, affecting lung parenchyma and the pleurae. Raised hyaline plaques may form in the parietal pleura, diaphragm, and pleura adjacent to the pericardium.

What to look for

Asbestosis causes numerous respiratory symptoms, including:
• dyspnea on exertion; possibly dyspnea at rest (with extensive fibrosis)
• severe, nonproductive cough (in nonsmokers); productive cough (in smokers)
• chest pain (usually pleuritic)
• pleural friction rub and crackles on auscultation
• decreased lung inflation
• decreased forced expiratory volume and vital capacity
• recurrent pleural effusions
• recurrent respiratory tract infections
• finger clubbing.

Asbestosis may progress to pulmonary fibrosis with respiratory failure and cardiovascular complications, including pulmonary hypertension and cor pulmonale.

What tests tell you

• Chest X-rays may show fine, irregular, linear, diffuse infiltrates. With extensive fibrosis, the lungs have a honeycomb or ground-glass appearance. Other findings include pleural thickening and calcification, bilateral obliteration

of costophrenic angles and, in later disease stages, an enlarged heart with a classic "shaggy" border.
• Pulmonary function tests (PFTs) may identify decreased vital capacity, forced vital capacity (FVC), and total lung capacity; decreased or normal forced expiratory volume in 1 second (FEV_1); a normal ratio of FEV_1 to FVC; and reduced diffusing capacity for carbon monoxide when fibrosis destroys alveolar walls and thickens the alveolocapillary membrane.
• ABG analysis may reveal decreased Pao_2 and $Paco_2$ from hyperventilation.

How it's treated

Treatment of asbestosis includes chest physiotherapy, aerosol therapy (including mucolytics), oxygen administration, and a high fluid intake of at least 3 qt (3 L) per day. Antibiotics are used to treat respiratory infections. Patients may also require diuretics, digoxin, and salt restriction.

What to do

Your care will be primarily supportive. Include the following measures in your care:
• Initiate measures to relieve symptoms and control complications.
• Provide chest physiotherapy as ordered.
• Administer antibiotics as ordered.
• Ensure adequate fluid intake and nutrition.
• Monitor the patient's sputum and provide frequent mouth care.

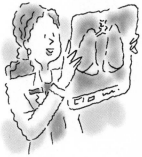

In a patient with extensive fibrosis, the lungs will have a honeycomb or ground-glass appearance on X-ray.

Asthma

Asthma is one type of COPD characterized by airflow resistance. Although asthma is a chronic reactive airway disorder, it may also present as an acute attack. Bronchospasms, increased mucus secretion, and mucosal edema cause episodic airway obstruction.

Battle of the sexes

Although asthma can strike at any age, about one-half of all patients are under age 10. In this age-group, twice as many boys as girls are affected. Furthermore, about one-

third of patients contract asthma between ages 10 and 30.
In this group, incidence is the same in both sexes.

It's all in the family

About one-third of all patients share the disease with at
least one immediate family member. Cases of asthma are
on the rise, prompting the National Institutes of Health to
initiate a study exploring possible causes of this increase.

What causes it

Extrinsic, or atopic, asthma is a sensitivity caused by specific external allergens, such as:
• pollen
• animal dander
• house dust or mold
• kapok or feather pillows
• food additives containing sulfites.
   Intrinsic, or nonatopic, asthma is a reaction to internal,
nonallergenic factors, such as:
• severe respiratory tract infection (especially in adults)
• irritants
• emotional stress
• fatigue
• endocrine changes
• temperature and humidity variations
• exposure to noxious fumes.
   Many asthmatics, especially children, have both intrinsic and extrinsic asthma.

Pathophysiology

In asthma, bronchial linings overreact to various stimuli, causing episodic smooth-muscle spasms that severely constrict the airways. Mucosal edema and thickened secretions further block the airways. (See *Understanding asthma.*)

What to look for

Signs and symptoms vary depending on the severity of
a patient's asthma.

On the mild side

Patients with mild asthma have adequate air exchange
and are asymptomatic between attacks. Signs and symp-

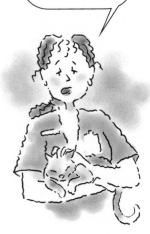

Don't jump
to conclusions.
Maybe it's stress,
and not you,
that's causing
my asthma to
flare up.

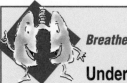

Breathe easy

Understanding asthma

Asthma is an inflammatory disease characterized by hyperresponsiveness of the airway and bronchospasm. These illustrations show the progression of an asthma attack.

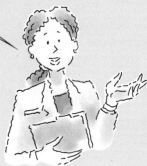

When the patient inhales a substance he's hypersensitive to, abnormal antibodies stimulate mast cells in the lung interstitium to release both histamine and slow-reacting substance of anaphylaxis.

Histamine stimulates the mucous membranes to secrete excessive mucus, further narrowing the bronchial lumen, as shown below.

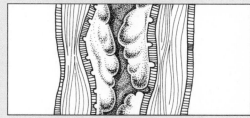

Histamine (H) attaches to receptor sites in the larger bronchi, where it causes swelling in smooth muscles.

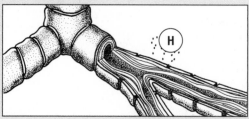

Slow-reacting substance of anaphylaxis (SRS-A) attaches to receptor sites in the smaller bronchi and causes swelling of smooth muscle there. SRS-A also causes fatty acids called *prostaglandins* to travel by way of the bloodstream to the lungs, where they enhance histamine's effects.

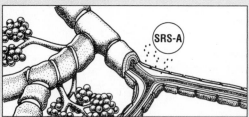

On inhalation, the narrowed bronchial lumen can still expand slightly, allowing air to reach the alveoli. On exhalation, increased intrathoracic pressure closes the bronchial lumen completely.

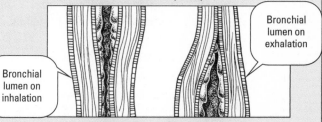

Bronchial lumen on inhalation

Bronchial lumen on exhalation

Mucus fills the lung bases, inhibiting alveolar ventilation, as shown below. Blood, shunted to alveoli in other lung parts, still can't compensate for diminished ventilation.

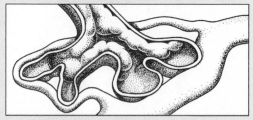

toms typically manifest after exposure to an allergen or trigger and include:
• brief episodes of wheezing, coughing, and dyspnea on exertion
• intermittent episodes of wheezing, coughing, and dyspnea (typically lasting less than 1 hour, once or twice per week).

Somewhere in the middle

Patients with moderate asthma have normal or below-normal air exchange as well as signs and symptoms that include:
• respiratory distress at rest
• hyperpnea (an abnormal increase in the depth and rate of respiration)
• exacerbations that last several days.

Under attack!

Patients may develop status asthmaticus, a severe attack that doesn't respond to conventional treatment. Signs and symptoms of this potentially life-threatening condition include:
• marked respiratory distress
• marked wheezing or absent breath sounds
• pulsus paradoxus greater than 10 mm Hg
• chest wall contractions.

What tests tell you

• PFTs reveal signs of airway obstructive disease, low-normal or decreased vital capacity, and increased total lung and residual capacities. Pulmonary function may be normal between attacks. PaO_2 and $PaCO_2$ are usually decreased, except in severe asthma, when $PaCO_2$ may be normal or increased, indicating severe bronchial obstruction.
• Serum immunoglobulin E levels may increase from an allergic reaction.
• CBC with differential reveals increased eosinophil count.
• Chest X-rays can diagnose or monitor asthma's progress and may show hyperinflation with areas of atelectasis.
• ABG analysis detects hypoxemia and guides treatment.

• Skin testing may identify specific allergens. Test results are read in 1 to 2 days to detect an early reaction and again after 4 to 5 days to reveal a late reaction.
• Bronchial challenge testing evaluates the clinical significance of allergens identified by skin testing.
• Pulse oximetry may show a reduced SaO_2 level.

How it's treated

Identifying and avoiding precipitating factors to prevent an asthma attack is the best treatment. If the stimuli can't be removed entirely, desensitization to specific antigens may be helpful.

Widening the roadway

Patients may also require treatment with bronchodilators to decrease bronchoconstriction, reduce bronchial airway edema, and increase pulmonary ventilation. Corticosteroids have the same effects as bronchodilators; they also have anti-inflammatory and immunosuppressive effects. Mast cell stabilizers block the acute obstructive effects of antigen exposure, thereby preventing the release of the chemical mediators responsible for anaphylaxis.

A breath of fresh air

If the patient is experiencing dyspnea, cyanosis, or hypoxemia, oxygen administration may be necessary. The amount delivered is designed to maintain the patient's PaO_2 between 65 and 85 mm Hg. Mechanical ventilation is needed if the patient doesn't respond to initial ventilatory support and drugs or develops respiratory failure.

What to do

Include the following measures when caring for the asthmatic patient:
• Perform careful, frequent assessments of the patient's respiratory status, including respiratory rate, breath sounds, and oxygen saturation levels.

Warning sign

• Take action when a patient with wheezes suddenly stops wheezing and continues to show signs of respiratory distress. The absence of wheezing may be due to bronchial constriction that narrows the airways severely. So little air passes through the narrowed airways that sound

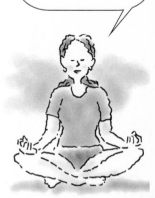

Alternative therapies such as yoga may help a patient recover from an asthma attack by increasing circulation.

is no longer produced. This is a sign of imminent respiratory collapse; the patient needs intubation and mechanical ventilation. Notify the doctor immediately, and remain with the patient.
• Assess the patient's mental status for confusion, agitation, or lethargy.
• Assess the patient's heart rate and rhythm. Monitor for cardiac arrhythmias related to bronchodilator therapy or hypoxemia.
• Administer medications and I.V. fluids as ordered.
• Position the patient for maximal comfort, and provide emotional support and reassurance.

Memory jogger

When you're with an asthmatic patient who suddenly takes a turn for the worse, use the acronym **RAP** to remember the signs of status asthmaticus:

Respiratory distress (marked changes in ability to breathe, increased wheezes, hyperventilation, chest retractions)

Absence of breath sounds (especially in a previously wheezing patient; indicates severe airway narrowing)

Pulsus paradoxus (greater than 10 mm Hg).

Atelectasis

Atelectasis, a condition marked by partial or total lung collapse and incomplete gas exchange, may be chronic or acute and commonly occurs to some degree in patients undergoing abdominal or thoracic surgery.

Get out of the way!

The prognosis depends on prompt removal of airway obstruction, relief of hypoxia, and reexpansion of the collapsed lobules or lung.

What causes it

Atelectasis may result from:
• bronchial occlusion by mucus plugs (a common problem in heavy smokers or people with COPD, bronchiectasis, or cystic fibrosis)
• occlusion by foreign bodies
• bronchogenic carcinoma
• inflammatory lung disease
• oxygen toxicity
• pulmonary edema
• any condition that inhibits full lung expansion or makes deep breathing painful, such as abdominal surgical incisions, rib fractures, tight dressings, and obesity
• prolonged immobility
• mechanical ventilation using constant small tidal volumes without intermittent deep breaths
• CNS depression (as in drug overdose), which eliminates periodic sighing.

Pathophysiology

In atelectasis, incomplete expansion of lobules (clusters of alveoli) or lung segments leads to partial or complete lung collapse.

Unfulfilling relationship

Because parts of the lung are unavailable for gas exchange, unoxygenated blood passes through these areas unchanged, resulting in hypoxemia.

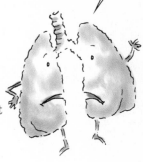

Hey, I'm headed for a collapse if you don't start aerating your lung bases!

What to look for

Your assessment findings will vary with the cause and degree of hypoxia and may include:
• dyspnea (possibly mild and subsiding without treatment if atelectasis involves only a small area of the lung, or severe if massive collapse occurs)
• cyanosis, decreased breath sounds
• anxiety and diaphoresis
• dull sound on percussion if a large portion of the lung is collapsed
• hypoxemia and tachycardia
• substernal or intercostal retraction
• compensatory hyperinflation of unaffected areas of the lung
• mediastinal shift to the affected side.

What tests tell you

• Chest X-rays show characteristic horizontal lines in the lower lung zones. Dense shadows accompany segmental or lobar collapse and are commonly associated with hyperinflation of neighboring lung zones during widespread atelectasis. Extensive areas of "micro-atelectasis" may exist, however, without showing abnormalities on the patient's chest X-ray.

Look out, we're going in!

• When the cause of atelectasis is unknown, bronchoscopy may be performed to rule out an obstructing neoplasm or a foreign body.

How it's treated

Atelectasis is treated with incentive spirometry, chest percussion, postural drainage, and frequent coughing and deep-breathing exercises.

Pipe cleaner

If these measures fail, bronchoscopy may help remove secretions. Humidity and bronchodilators can improve mucociliary clearance and dilate airways and are sometimes used with a nebulizer. Atelectasis secondary to an obstructing neoplasm may require surgery or radiation therapy.

What to do

Your goal is to keep the patient's airways clear and relieve hypoxia. To achieve this, follow these guidelines:
• To prevent atelectasis, encourage the patient to cough, turn, and breathe deeply every 1 to 2 hours as ordered. Teach the patient to splint his incision when coughing. Gently reposition a postoperative patient often, and help him walk as soon as possible. Administer adequate analgesics to control pain.

Heavy sighing

• During mechanical ventilation, tidal volume should be maintained at 10 to 15 ml/kg of the patient's body weight to ensure adequate lung expansion. Use the sigh mechanism on the ventilator, if appropriate, to intermittently increase tidal volume at the rate of three to four sighs per hour.
• Humidify inspired air and encourage adequate fluid intake to mobilize secretions. Loosen and clear secretions with postural drainage and chest percussion.
• Assess breath sounds and ventilatory status frequently and report changes.
• Evaluate the patient. Secretions should be clear and the patient should show no signs of hypoxia. (See *Teaching the patient with atelectasis.*)

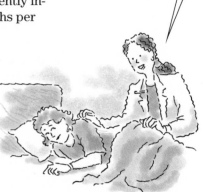

Making sure your patient coughs, turns, and deep-breathes every 1 to 2 hours is crucial for preventing atelectasis.

> ## Teaching the patient with atelectasis
>
> Teach the patient how to use an incentive spirometer. Encourage him to use it for 10 to 20 breaths every hour while he's awake. Also, teach him about respiratory care, including postural drainage, coughing, and deep breathing.
>
> Encourage the patient to stop smoking and lose weight as needed. Refer him to appropriate support groups for help. Because the patient may be frightened by his limited breathing capacity, provide reassurance and emotional support.

Bronchiectasis

An irreversible condition marked by chronic abnormal dilation of bronchi and destruction of bronchial walls, bronchiectasis can occur throughout the tracheobronchial tree or can be confined to one segment or lobe.

An equal opportunity disorder

However, bronchiectasis is usually bilateral, involving the basilar segments of the lower lobes. It affects people of both sexes and all ages.

What causes it

Bronchiectasis may be caused by such conditions as:
- mucoviscidosis (cystic fibrosis of the pancreas)
- immunologic disorders such as agammaglobulinemia
- recurrent, inadequately treated bacterial respiratory tract infections such as TB
- measles, pneumonia, pertussis, or influenza
- obstruction by a foreign body, tumor, or stenosis associated with recurrent infection
- inhalation of corrosive gas or repeated aspiration of gastric juices into the lungs.

Pathophysiology

Bronchiectasis results from repeated damage to bronchial walls and abnormal mucociliary clearance that causes breakdown of supportive tissue adjacent to the airways. This disease has three forms: cylindrical (fusiform), varicose, and saccular (cystic). (See *Forms of bronchiectasis*, page 152.)

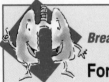

Breathe easy

Forms of bronchiectasis

The different forms of bronchiectasis may occur separately or simultaneously. In *cylindrical* bronchiectasis, the bronchi expand unevenly, with little change in diameter, and end suddenly in a squared-off fashion. In *varicose* bronchiectasis, abnormal, irregular dilation and narrowing of the bronchi give the appearance of varicose veins. In *saccular* bronchiectasis, many large dilations end in sacs. These sacs balloon into pus-filled cavities as they approach the periphery and are then called *saccules.*

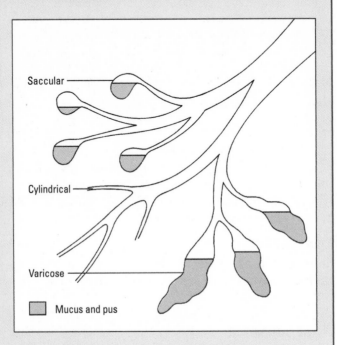

Saccular

Cylindrical

Varicose

☐ Mucus and pus

What to look for

Initially, bronchiectasis may not produce symptoms. Assess your patient for a chronic cough that produces copious, foul-smelling, mucopurulent secretions, possibly totaling several cupfuls daily (classic symptom). Other characteristic findings include:
- coarse crackles during inspiration over involved lobes or segments
- occasional wheezes
- dyspnea
- weight loss and malaise
- clubbing of fingers and toes
- recurrent fever, chills, and other signs of infection.

What tests tell you

In addition to aiding diagnosis, the following tests also help determine the physiologic severity of the disease and the effects of therapy and help evaluate the patient for surgery:
• Bronchography is the most reliable diagnostic test and reveals the location and extent of disease.
• Chest X-rays show peribronchial thickening, areas of atelectasis, and scattered cystic changes.
• Bronchoscopy helps identify the source of secretions or the site of bleeding in hemoptysis.
• Sputum culture and Gram stain identify predominant organisms.
• CBC and WBC differential identify anemia and leukocytosis.
• PFTs detect decreased vital capacity and decreased expiratory flow.
• ABG analysis shows hypoxemia.

How it's treated

Patients with bronchiectasis typically receive antibiotics by mouth or I.V. for 7 to 10 days or until sputum production decreases. If the patient has bronchospasm and thick, tenacious sputum, bronchodilators may be given along with postural drainage and chest percussion to help remove secretions. Occasionally, bronchoscopy may be used to aid removal of secretions.

The patient may also require oxygen therapy to treat hypoxemia. If hemoptysis is severe, lobectomy or segmental resection may be performed.

What to do

Care is primarily supportive. Incorporate the following measures into a care plan:
• Provide a warm, quiet, comfortable environment and urge the patient to rest as much as possible.
• Administer antibiotics as ordered.

Chest PT — first and last

• Perform chest physiotherapy several times per day (early morning and bedtime are best); include postural drainage and chest percussion for involved lobes. Have

Teaching the patient with bronchiectasis

When caring for a patient with bronchiectasis, be sure to explain all diagnostic tests. Advise the patient to stop smoking, which stimulates secretions and irritates the airways, and refer him to a local self-help group.

Show family members how to perform postural drainage and percussion. Also, teach the patient coughing and deep-breathing techniques to promote good ventilation and the removal of secretions. Teach the patient how to properly dispose of secretions.

Caution the patient to avoid air pollutants and people with upper respiratory tract infections. Instruct him to take medications (especially antibiotics) exactly as ordered. To help prevent this disease, vigorously treat bacterial pneumonia and stress the need for immunization to prevent childhood diseases.

the patient maintain each position for 10 minutes; then perform percussion and tell him to cough.
• Encourage balanced, high-protein meals to promote good health and tissue healing and plenty of fluids to aid expectoration.
• Provide frequent mouth care to remove foul-smelling sputum.
• Evaluate the patient. His secretions should be thin and clear or white. (See *Teaching the patient with bronchiectasis.*)

Chronic obstructive pulmonary disease

COPD is an umbrella term that may refer to emphysema, chronic bronchitis, asthma and, more commonly, any combination of these conditions (usually bronchitis and emphysema). The most common chronic lung disease, COPD affects an estimated 30 million U.S. residents, and its incidence is rising. It now ranks third among the major causes of death in the United States.

Where there's smoke there's...COPD

COPD affects more men than women, probably because until recently men were more likely to smoke heavily. However, the rate of COPD among women is increasing. Early COPD may not produce symptoms and may cause only

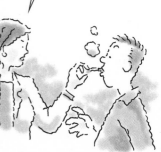

Don't you know that smoking is a major cause of COPD?

minimal disability in many patients, but it tends to worsen with time.

What causes it

COPD may be caused by:
- cigarette smoking
- recurrent or chronic respiratory tract infection
- allergies
- familial and hereditary factors such as $alpha_1$-antitrypsin deficiency.

Pathophysiology

Smoking, one of the major causes of COPD, impairs ciliary action and macrophage function and causes inflammation in the airways, increased mucus production, destruction of alveolar septa, and peribronchiolar fibrosis. Early inflammatory changes may reverse if the patient stops smoking before lung disease becomes extensive.

Clogging up the system

The mucus plugs and narrowed airways cause air trapping, as in chronic bronchitis and emphysema. Hyperinflation of the alveoli occurs on expiration. On inspiration, airways enlarge, allowing air to pass beyond the obstruction; on expiration, airways narrow, preventing gas flow. Air trapping (also called *ball valving)* occurs commonly in asthma and chronic bronchitis.

What to look for

The typical patient with COPD is asymptomatic until middle age, when the following signs and symptoms may occur:
- reduced ability to exercise or do strenuous work
- productive cough
- dyspnea with minimal exertion
- diminished, low-pitched breath sounds
- sonorous or sibilant wheezes (or both)
- prolonged expiration
- fine, inspiratory crackles.

What tests tell you

- In advanced disease, a chest X-ray reveals a flattened diaphragm, reduced vascular markings at the lung periph-

ery, hyperinflation of the lungs, a vertical heart, enlarged anteroposterior chest diameter, and a large retrosternal air space.
• PFTs show increased residual volume, total lung capacity, and compliance as well as decreased vital capacity, diffusing capacity, and expiratory volumes.
• ABG analysis indicates a reduced PaO_2 with normal $PaCO_2$ until late in the disease.
• At later stages, an ECG will reveal signs of right ventricular hypertrophy, such as tall, symmetrical P waves in leads II, III, and aV_F; and vertical QRS axis.
• Late in the disease when persistent severe hypoxia is present, a red blood cell (RBC) count will show increased hemoglobin levels.

How it's treated

Treatment for COPD aims to relieve symptoms and prevent complications. Most patients receive beta-adrenergic agonist bronchodilators (albuterol or salmeterol), anticholinergic bronchodilators (ipratropium), and corticosteroids (beclomethasone or triamcinolone). These drugs are usually given by metered-dose inhaler.

What to do

Your care should include these measures:
• Administer antibiotics, as ordered, to treat respiratory tract infections.
• Administer low concentrations of oxygen as ordered.
• Check ABG levels regularly to determine oxygen need and to avoid carbon dioxide narcosis.
• Evaluate the patient. The patient's chest X-rays, respiratory rate and rhythm, ABG values, and pH should be normal. PaO_2 should be greater than 60 mm Hg. Body weight and urine output should also be normal. (See *Teaching the patient with COPD*.)

Cor pulmonale

In cor pulmonale, or right ventricular hypertrophy, the ventricle enlarges and dilates at the end stage of a disease that affects the structure, function, or vasculature of the lungs, in some cases resulting in heart failure. It doesn't

Teaching the patient with COPD

Familiarize the patient with prescribed bronchodilators. Explain that bronchodilators alleviate bronchospasm and enhance mucociliary clearance of secretions. Teach or reinforce the correct method of using an inhaler.

To strengthen the muscles of respiration, teach the patient to take slow, deep breaths and exhale through pursed lips. Teach him how to cough effectively to help mobilize secretions. If secretions are thick, urge the patient to drink 12 to 15 glasses of fluid per day.

Urge the patient to stop smoking and to avoid other respiratory irritants. Suggest that an air conditioner with an air filter may prove helpful. If the patient is to continue oxygen therapy at home, teach him how to use the equipment correctly.

occur, however, with disorders stemming from congenital heart disease or those affecting the left side of the heart.

Familiar relationship

About 85% of patients with cor pulmonale also have COPD, and about 25% of patients with bronchial COPD eventually develop cor pulmonale. It's most common in smokers and in middle-aged and elderly men; however, the incidence in women is rising.

What causes it

Cor pulmonale may result from:
- disorders that affect the pulmonary parenchyma
- pulmonary diseases that affect the airways (such as COPD and bronchial asthma)
- vascular diseases (such as vasculitis, pulmonary emboli, or external vascular obstruction from a tumor or aneurysm)
- chest wall abnormalities (such as kyphoscoliosis and pectus excavatum [funnel chest])
- neuromuscular disorders (such as muscular dystrophy and poliomyelitis)
- external factors (such as obesity or living at a high altitude).

Pathophysiology

In cor pulmonale, pulmonary hypertension increases the heart's workload. To compensate, the right ventricle hypertrophies to force blood through the lungs. As long as the heart can compensate for the increased pulmonary vascular resistance, signs and symptoms reflect only the underlying disorder.

What to look for

In early stages of cor pulmonale, patients are most likely to report:
- chronic productive cough
- exertional dyspnea
- wheezing respirations
- fatigue and weakness.

When I encounter resistance from the lungs, my right side has to work harder, which causes my right ventricle to enlarge.

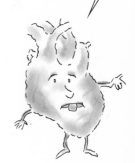

Filling up the place

As the compensatory mechanism begins to fail, larger amounts of blood remain in the right ventricle at the end of diastole, causing ventricular dilation. As cor pulmonale progresses, these additional symptoms occur:
• dyspnea at rest
• tachypnea
• orthopnea
• dependent edema
• distended neck veins
• enlarged, tender liver
• hepatojugular reflux (distention of the jugular vein induced by pressing over the liver)
• right upper quadrant discomfort
• tachycardia
• decreased cardiac output.

Chest examination reveals characteristics of the underlying lung disease.

When the solution is part of the problem

In response to hypoxia, the bone marrow produces more RBCs, causing polycythemia. The blood's viscosity increases, which further aggravates pulmonary hypertension. This increases the right ventricle's workload, causing heart failure.

Eventually, cor pulmonale may lead to biventricular failure, hepatomegaly, edema, ascites, and pleural effusions. Polycythemia increases the risk of thromboembolism. Because cor pulmonale occurs late in the course of COPD and other irreversible diseases, the prognosis is poor. (See *Understanding cor pulmonale.*)

What tests tell you

The following tests are used to diagnose cor pulmonale:
• PA catheterization shows increased right ventricular and PA pressures, resulting from increased pulmonary vascular resistance. Both right ventricular systolic and pulmonary artery systolic pressures are above 30 mm Hg, and pulmonary artery diastolic pressure is higher than 15 mm Hg.
• Echocardiography or angiography demonstrates right ventricular enlargement.

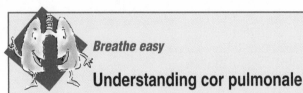

Breathe easy

Understanding cor pulmonale

Three types of disorders are responsible for cor pulmonale:

1 pulmonary restrictive disorders, such as fibrosis or obesity

2 pulmonary obstructive disorders, such as bronchitis

3 primary vascular disorders, such as recurrent pulmonary emboli.

These disorders share a common pathway to the formation of cor pulmonale. Hypoxic constriction of pulmonary blood vessels and obstruction of pulmonary blood flow lead to increased pulmonary resistance, which progresses to cor pulmonale.

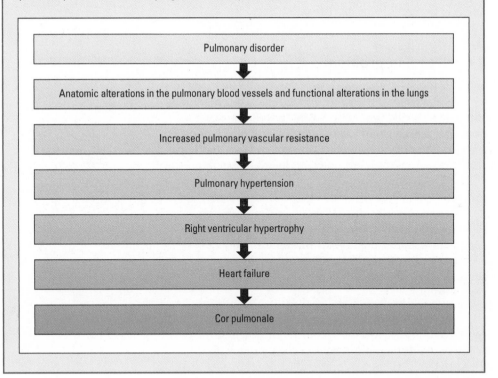

Pulmonary disorder

↓

Anatomic alterations in the pulmonary blood vessels and functional alterations in the lungs

↓

Increased pulmonary vascular resistance

↓

Pulmonary hypertension

↓

Right ventricular hypertrophy

↓

Heart failure

↓

Cor pulmonale

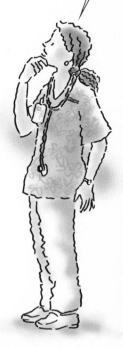

Three types of disorders may cause cor pulmonale, but all share a common pathway.

• Chest X-rays reveal large central pulmonary arteries and right ventricular enlargement.
• ABG analysis detects decreased Pao_2 (usually less than 70 mm Hg and never more than 90 mm Hg).

- Pulse oximetry shows a reduced Sao_2 level.
- ECG discloses arrhythmias, such as premature atrial and ventricular contractions and atrial fibrillation during severe hypoxia. It may also show right bundle-branch block, right axis deviation, prominent P waves, and an inverted T wave in right precordial leads.
- PFTs reflect underlying pulmonary disease.
- Magnetic resonance imaging measures right ventricular mass, wall thickness, and ejection fraction.
- Cardiac catheterization measures pulmonary vascular pressures.
- Hematocrit is typically over 50%.
- Serum liver enzyme levels show an elevated level of aspartate aminotransferase with hepatic congestion and decreased liver function.
- Serum bilirubin levels may be elevated if liver dysfunction and hepatomegaly are present.

How it's treated

Treatment for cor pulmonale aims to reduce hypoxemia and pulmonary vasoconstriction, increase exercise tolerance, and correct underlying conditions. Treatment measures include bed rest, antibiotics for respiratory infections, pulmonary artery vasodilators, and continuous administration of low concentrations of oxygen. Patients should also receive a low-sodium diet and restricted fluids.

Rest is part of the solution for right ventricular hypertrophy.

Blood sucker

Phlebotomy, to decrease RBC mass, along with anticoagulation using small doses of heparin, may decrease the risk of thromboembolism. In cases of acute disease, the patient may require mechanical ventilation.

What to do

When caring for a patient with cor pulmonale, follow these steps:
- Make sure that the patient receives a low-sodium diet.
- Monitor the patient's fluid intake.
- Administer antibiotics and vasodilators as ordered.
- Administer oxygen as ordered.
- Monitor the patient's respiratory status.

Heart failure

When the myocardium can't pump effectively enough to meet the body's metabolic needs, heart failure occurs. Pump failure usually occurs in a damaged left ventricle, but may also happen in the right ventricle. Usually, left-sided heart failure develops first. Heart failure is classified as:
- acute or chronic
- left-sided or right-sided (see *Understanding left- and right-sided heart failure*, pages 162 and 163.)
- systolic or diastolic. (See *Classifying heart failure*, page 164.)

Quality time

Although symptoms of heart failure may restrict the patient's ability to perform normal activities of daily living (ADLs) and severely affect his quality of life, advances in diagnostic and therapeutic techniques have greatly improved patient outcome. However, prognosis still depends on the underlying cause and its response to treatment.

What causes it

Cardiovascular disorders that lead to heart failure include:
- atherosclerotic heart disease
- MI
- hypertension
- rheumatic heart disease
- congenital heart disease
- ischemic heart disease
- cardiomyopathy
- valvular diseases
- arrhythmias.
   Noncardiovascular causes of heart failure include:
- pregnancy and childbirth
- increased environmental temperature or humidity
- severe physical or mental stress
- thyrotoxicosis
- acute blood loss
- pulmonary embolism
- severe infection
- COPD.

Breathe easy

Understanding left- and right-sided heart failure

These illustrations show how myocardial damage leads to heart failure.

Left-sided heart failure

Increased workload and end-diastolic volume enlarge the left ventricle (see illustration below). Because of lack of oxygen, the ventricle enlarges with stretched tissue rather than functional tissue. The patient may experience increased heart rate, pale and cool skin, tingling in the extremities, decreased cardiac output, and arrhythmias.

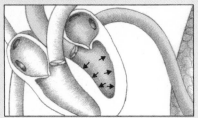

Diminished left ventricular function allows blood to pool in the ventricle and the atrium and eventually back up into the pulmonary veins and capillaries (as shown below). At this stage, the patient may experience dyspnea on exertion, confusion, dizziness, orthostatic hypotension, decreased peripheral pulses and pulse pressure, cyanosis, and an S_3 gallop.

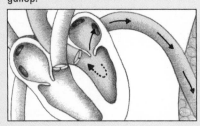

As the pulmonary circulation becomes engorged, rising capillary pressure pushes sodium (Na) and water (H_2O) into the interstitial space (as shown below), causing pulmonary edema. You'll note coughing, subclavian retractions, crackles, tachypnea, elevated pulmonary artery pressure, diminished pulmonary compliance, and increased partial pressure of carbon dioxide.

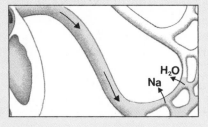

$$H_2O$$
$$Na$$

When the patient lies down, fluid in the extremities moves into the systemic circulation. Because the left ventricle can't handle the increased venous return, fluid pools in the pulmonary circulation, worsening pulmonary edema (see illustration below). You may note decreased breath sounds, dullness on percussion, crackles, and orthopnea.

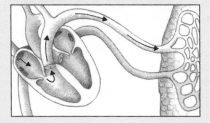

The right ventricle may now become stressed because it's pumping against greater pulmonary vascular resistance and left ventricular pressure (see illustration below). When this occurs, the patient's symptoms worsen.

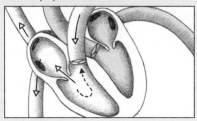

Right-sided heart failure

The stressed right ventricle enlarges with the formation of stretched tissue (see illustration below). Increasing conduction time and deviation of the heart from its normal axis can cause arrhythmias. If the patient doesn't already have left-sided heart failure, he may experience increased heart rate, cool skin, cyanosis, decreased cardiac output, palpitations, and dyspnea.

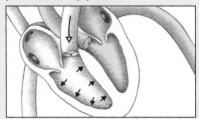

Understanding left- and right-sided heart failure *(continued)*

Blood pools in the right ventricle and right atrium. The backed-up blood causes pressure and congestion in the vena cava and systemic circulation (see illustration below). The patient will have elevated central venous pressure, jugular vein distention, and hepatojugular reflux.

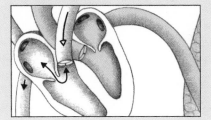

Backed-up blood also distends the visceral veins, especially the hepatic vein. As the liver and spleen become engorged (see illustration below), their function is impaired. The patient may develop anorexia, nausea, abdominal pain, palpable liver and spleen, weakness, and dyspnea secondary to abdominal distention.

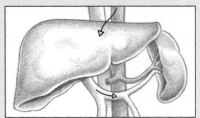

Rising capillary pressure forces excess fluid from the capillaries into the interstitial space (see illustration below). This causes tissue edema, especially in the lower extremities and abdomen. The patient may experience weight gain, pitting edema, and nocturia.

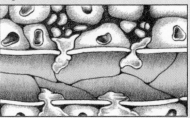

Pathophysiology

The patient's underlying condition determines whether heart failure is acute or insidious. Heart failure is commonly associated with systolic or diastolic overloading and myocardial weakness. As stress on the heart muscle reaches a critical level, the muscle's contractility is reduced and cardiac output declines. Venous input to the ventricle remains the same, however.

A heartfelt response

The body's responses to decreased cardiac output include:
• a reflex increase in sympathetic activity
• the release of renin from the juxtaglomerular cells of the kidney
• anaerobic metabolism by affected cells
• increased extraction of oxygen by the peripheral cells.

Classifying heart failure

Heart failure is classified according to its pathophysiology. It may be left- or right-sided, systolic or diastolic, and acute or chronic.

Right-sided or left-sided

Right-sided heart failure results from ineffective right ventricular contraction. Although acute right ventricular infarction or pulmonary embolus may cause right-sided heart failure, the most common cause is profound backward flow due to left-sided heart failure.

In contrast, *left-sided heart failure* results from ineffective left ventricular contraction. Common causes of left-sided heart failure include left ventricular myocardial infarction, hypertension, and aortic and mitral valve stenosis or insufficiency. As the decreased pumping ability of the left ventricle persists, fluid accumulates, backing up into the left atrium and then into the lungs. If this worsens, pulmonary edema and right-sided heart failure may also result.

Systolic or diastolic

In *systolic heart failure*, the left ventricle fails to pump out enough blood to the systemic circulation during systole. The ejection fraction falls, causing blood to back up into the pulmonary circulation. In turn, the pressure in the pulmonary venous system rises, and cardiac output falls.

In *diastolic heart failure*, the left ventricle fails to relax and fill properly during diastole. Stroke volume falls. As a result, larger ventricular volumes are needed to maintain cardiac output.

Acute or chronic

The term *acute* refers to the timing of the onset of symptoms and also to whether compensatory mechanisms have occurred. In *acute heart failure*, the patient's fluid status is usually normal or low. Also, the patient doesn't retain sodium or water.

In *chronic heart failure,* the patient's signs and symptoms have been evident for some time and compensatory mechanisms are well established. Although the patient typically has persistent fluid volume overload, drugs, diet changes, and activity restrictions usually help to control symptoms.

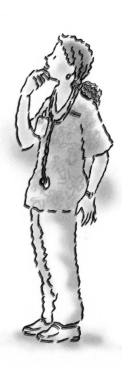

Adept at adaptation

When blood in the ventricles increases, the heart compensates, or adapts. Compensation may occur for long periods before signs and symptoms develop.

Adaptations may be short-term or long-term. As a short-term adaptation, the length of the heart's end-diastolic fibers increases. In response, the ventricular muscle dilates and increases the force of contractions. (This is called the *Frank-Starling curve*.) A long-term adaptation occurs when ventricular hypertrophy increases the heart muscle's ability to contract and push its volume of blood into circulation.

> Your left ventricle looks enlarged. You've obviously been compensating for quite some time.

What to look for

Clinical signs of left-sided heart failure include:
• dyspnea (initially upon exertion, also paroxysmal nocturnal)
• Cheyne-Stokes respirations
• cough
• orthopnea
• bibasilar crackles
• tachycardia
• ventricular gallop (heard over the apex)
• fatigue
• muscle weakness
• edema and weight gain
• irritability
• restlessness
• shortened attention span.
    The patient with right-sided heart failure may develop:
• edema, initially dependent
• jugular vein distention
• hepatomegaly.

What tests tell you

• Blood tests may show elevated blood urea nitrogen (BUN) and creatinine levels, elevated serum norepinephrine levels, and elevated transaminase and bilirubin levels if hepatic function is impaired.
• Elevated blood levels of brain natriuretic peptide may correctly identify heart failure in as many as 83% of patients.

• ECG reflects heart strain or ventricular enlargement (ischemia). It may also reveal atrial enlargement, tachycardia, and extrasystoles, suggesting heart failure.
• Chest X-rays show increased pulmonary vascular markings, interstitial edema, or pleural effusion and cardiomegaly.
• Multiple-gated acquisition scan shows a decreased ejection fraction in left-sided heart failure.
• Cardiac catheterization may show ventricular dilation, coronary artery occlusion, and valvular disorders (such as aortic stenosis) in both left- and right-sided heart failure.
• Echocardiography may show ventricular hypertrophy, decreased contractility, and valvular disorders in both left- and right-sided heart failure. Serial echocardiograms may help assess the patient's response to therapy.
• Cardiopulmonary exercise testing to evaluate the patient's ventricular performance during exercise may show decreased oxygen uptake.

How it's treated

Measures include diuretics that reduce preload by decreasing total blood volume and circulatory congestion. Angiotensin-converting enzyme (ACE) inhibitors dilate blood vessels and decrease systemic vascular resistance, thereby reducing the heart's workload. Vasodilators may be given to the patient who can't tolerate ACE inhibitors. Vasodilators increase cardiac output by reducing impedance to ventricular outflow, thereby decreasing afterload.

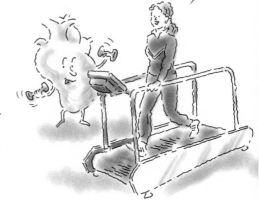

One way to test for heart failure is to have your patient perform cardiopulmonary exercise to evaluate his ventricular performance.

Pump it up

Digoxin may help strengthen myocardial contractility. Beta-adrenergic blockers may prevent cardiac remodeling (left ventricular dilation and hypertrophy). Nesiritide, a human B-type natriuretic peptide, may be administered to augment diuresis and to decrease afterload. Positive inotropic agents, such as I.V. dopamine or dobutamine, are reserved for those with end-stage heart failure or those awaiting heart transplantation.

Break time

The patient must alternate periods of rest with periods of activity and follow a sodium-restricted diet with smaller, more frequent meals. He may have to wear antiembolism stockings to prevent venostasis and possible thromboembolism formation. The doctor may also order oxygen therapy.

On the cutting edge

Although controversial, surgery may be performed if the patient's heart failure doesn't improve after therapy and lifestyle modifications. If the patient with valve dysfunction has recurrent acute heart failure, he may undergo surgical valve replacement. Coronary artery bypass grafting, percutaneous transluminal coronary angioplasty, or stenting may be performed in a patient with heart failure caused by ischemia.

In some cases, a partial left ventriculectomy, or *ventricular remodeling*, may be performed to remove nonviable heart muscle, thereby reducing the size of the hypertrophied ventricle and allowing the heart to pump more efficiently. Patients with severe heart failure may benefit from a mechanical ventricular assist device or heart transplantation. An internal cardioverter-defibrillator may be implanted to treat life-threatening arrhythmias. A biventricular pacemaker may be placed to control ventricular dyssynchrony.

What to do

When caring for a patient with heart failure, be sure to incorporate the following into your care plan:
• Frequently monitor BUN, serum creatinine, potassium, sodium, chloride, and magnesium levels.
• Reinforce the importance of adhering to the prescribed diet. If fluid restrictions have been ordered, arrange a mutually acceptable schedule for allowable fluids.
• Weigh the patient daily to assess for fluid overload.
• To prevent deep vein thrombosis from vascular congestion, assist the patient with range-of-motion (ROM) exercises. Enforce bed rest, and apply antiembolism stockings. Watch for calf pain and tenderness. Organize activities to ensure adequate rest periods.
• Evaluate the patient. Successful recovery should reveal clear lungs, normal heart sounds, adequate blood pressure, and absence of dyspnea or edema. The patient should be able to perform ADLs and maintain his normal weight. (See *Teaching the patient with heart failure,* page 168.)

> Successful recovery from heart failure reveals clear lungs, normal heart sounds, adequate blood pressure, and absence of dyspnea or edema.

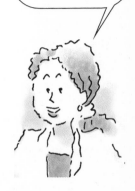

> ## Teaching the patient with heart failure
>
> When caring for a patient with heart failure, teach him about lifestyle changes. Advise him to avoid foods high in sodium to help curb fluid overload. Explain that the potassium he loses through diuretic therapy must be replaced by a prescribed potassium supplement and eating high-potassium foods.
>
> Stress the need for regular checkups and the benefits of balancing activity and rest. Also reinforce the importance of taking cardiac glycosides exactly as prescribed. Caution the patient to watch for and report signs of toxicity.
>
> Tell the patient to notify the doctor if he experiences any of these signs or symptoms:
> * an unusually irregular pulse, or a pulse rate under 60 beats/minute
> * dizziness, blurred vision, shortness of breath, paroxysmal nocturnal dyspnea, swollen ankles, or decreased urine output
> * weight gain of 3 to 5 lb (1.5 to 2.5 kg) in 1 week.

Pleural effusion

Pleural effusion is an excess of fluid in the pleural space. Normally, this space contains a small amount of extracellular fluid that lubricates the pleural surfaces. Increased production or inadequate removal of this fluid results in transudative or exudative pleural effusion. Empyema, the accumulation of pus and necrotic tissue in the pleural space, is also a form of pleural effusion.

What causes it

Transudative pleural effusion can stem from:
* heart failure
* hepatic disease with ascites
* peritoneal dialysis
* hypoalbuminemia
* disorders resulting in overexpanded intravascular volume.

Follow all exit signs, please

Exudative pleural effusion can stem from:
* TB
* subphrenic abscess

- esophageal rupture
- pancreatitis
- bacterial or fungal pneumonitis
- empyema
- cancer
- pulmonary embolism with or without infarction
- collagen disorders (such as lupus erythematosus and rheumatoid arthritis)
- myxedema
- chest trauma.

Pathophysiology

In transudative pleural effusion, excessive hydrostatic pressure or decreased osmotic pressure allows excessive fluid to pass across intact capillaries, resulting in an ultra-filtrate of plasma containing low concentrations of protein.

Leaky pipes

In exudative pleural effusion, capillaries exhibit increased permeability, with or without changes in hydrostatic and colloid osmotic pressures, allowing protein-rich fluid to leak into the pleural space. Empyema is usually associated with infection in the pleural space.

What to look for

Assess your patient for the following signs and symptoms:
- dyspnea
- dry cough
- pleural friction rub
- possible pleuritic pain that worsens with coughing or deep breathing
- dullness on percussion
- tachycardia
- tachypnea
- decreased chest motion and breath sounds.

What tests tell you

Examination of pleural fluid obtained by thoracentesis reveals these findings:
- In transudative effusions, specific gravity is usually less than 1.015 and protein less than 3 g/dl.

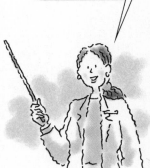

Remember, in transudative pleural effusion, fluid passes through intact capillaries because of a change in hydrostatic or osmotic pressures. In exudative pleural effusion, capillaries have increased permeability and "exude" fluid.

- In exudative effusions, specific gravity is greater than 1.02, and the ratio of protein in pleural fluid to serum is equal to or greater than 0.5. Pleural fluid lactate dehydrogenase (LD) is equal to or greater than 200 IU, and the ratio of LD in pleural fluid to LD in serum is equal to or greater than 0.6.
- If a pleural effusion results from esophageal rupture or pancreatitis, amylase levels in aspirated fluid are usually higher than serum levels.
- In empyema, cell analysis shows leukocytosis.
- Aspirated fluid may also be tested for lupus erythematosus cells, antinuclear antibodies, and neoplastic cells. It may be analyzed for color and consistency; acid-fast bacillus, fungal, and bacterial cultures; and triglycerides (in chylothorax).
- Chest X-ray shows radiopaque fluid in dependent regions.
- Pleural biopsy may be particularly useful for confirming TB or cancer.

How it's treated

Depending on the amount of fluid present, symptomatic effusion requires either thoracentesis to remove fluid or careful monitoring of the patient's own fluid reabsorption. Hemothorax requires drainage to prevent fibrothorax formation. Associated hypoxia requires supplemental oxygen.

What to do

Implement the following measures as part of your care:
- Administer oxygen as ordered.
- Provide meticulous chest tube care and use sterile technique for changing dressings around the tube insertion site in empyema. Record the amount, color, and consistency of tube drainage.
- If the patient has open drainage through a rib resection or an intercostal tube, follow standard precautions. Because weeks of such drainage are usually necessary to obliterate the space, make visiting nurse referrals for patients who will be discharged with the tube in place.
- If pleural effusion was a complication of pneumonia or influenza, advise the patient to seek prompt medical attention for chest colds.

• Evaluate the patient. He should remain afebrile and have minimal chest discomfort and a normal respiratory pattern. (See *Teaching the patient with pleural effusion.*)

Pneumonia

Pneumonia is an acute infection of the lung parenchyma that commonly impairs gas exchange. The prognosis is usually good for people who have normal lungs and adequate host defenses before the onset of pneumonia; however, bacterial pneumonia is the fifth leading cause of death in debilitated patients. The disorder occurs in primary and secondary forms.

What causes it

Pneumonia is caused by an infecting pathogen (bacterial or viral) or by a chemical or other irritant (such as aspirated material). Certain predisposing factors increase the risk of pneumonia.

For bacterial and viral pneumonia, these include:
• chronic illness and debilitation
• cancer (particularly lung cancer)
• abdominal and thoracic surgery
• atelectasis, aspiration
• colds or other viral respiratory infections
• chronic respiratory disease, such as COPD, asthma, bronchiectasis, and cystic fibrosis
• smoking, alcoholism
• malnutrition
• sickle cell disease
• tracheostomy
• exposure to noxious gases
• immunosuppressive therapy.

Aspiring to be risky

Aspiration pneumonia is more likely to occur in elderly or debilitated patients, those receiving nasogastric (NG) tube feedings, and those with an impaired gag reflex, poor oral hygiene, or a decreased LOC. (See *Pneumonia in older adults*, page 172.)

Teaching the patient with pleural effusion

Teach the patient what to expect in a thoracentesis. Reassure him during the procedure and observe for complications.

Encourage the patient to perform deep-breathing exercises to promote lung expansion and to use an incentive spirometer to promote deep breathing.

Bacterial pneumonia is the fifth leading cause of death in debilitated patients. Take every precaution to help prevent this infection from occurring.

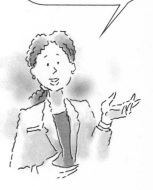

Pathophysiology

In general, the lower respiratory tract can be exposed to pathogens by inhalation, aspiration, vascular dissemination, or direct contact with contaminated equipment such as suction catheters. After pathogens are inside, they begin to colonize and infection develops.

Getting bogged down

In bacterial pneumonia, which can occur in any part of the lungs, an infection initially triggers alveolar inflammation and edema. This produces an area of low ventilation with normal perfusion. Capillaries become engorged with blood, causing stasis. As the alveolar capillary membrane breaks down, alveoli fill with blood and exudate, resulting in atelectasis. In severe bacterial infections, the lungs look heavy and liverlike — similar to ARDS.

Attacking on the way in

In viral pneumonia, the virus first attacks bronchiolar epithelial cells. This causes interstitial inflammation and desquamation. The virus also invades bronchial mucous glands and goblet cells. It then spreads to the alveoli, which fill with blood and fluid.

Caustic response

In aspiration pneumonia, inhalation of gastric juices or hydrocarbons triggers inflammatory changes and inactivates surfactant over a large area. Decreased surfactant leads to alveolar collapse. Acidic gastric juices may damage the airways and alveoli. Particles containing aspirated gastric juices may obstruct the airways and reduce airflow, leading to secondary bacterial pneumonia.

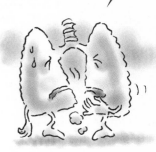

I have a productive cough, I hurt, and I have fever and chills. What does that tell you?

What to look for

The five cardinal signs and symptoms of early bacterial pneumonia are:

 coughing

 sputum production

 pleuritic chest pain

 shaking chills

 fever.

Other signs vary widely, ranging from diffuse, fine crackles to signs of localized or extensive consolidation and pleural effusion.

What tests tell you

• Chest X-rays showing infiltrates and a sputum smear demonstrating acute inflammatory cells support the diagnosis.
• Positive blood cultures in patients with pulmonary infiltrates strongly suggest pneumonia produced by the organisms isolated from the blood cultures.
• Occasionally, a transtracheal aspirate of tracheobronchial secretions or bronchoscopy with brushings may be performed to obtain material for smear and culture.
• Early *Pneumocystis carinii* pneumonia can be detected only by a $\dot{V}/\dot{Q}$ scan.

How it's treated

Antimicrobial therapy varies with the infecting agent. Therapy should be reevaluated early in the course of treatment.

Lending support

Supportive measures include humidified oxygen therapy for hypoxemia, mechanical ventilation for respiratory failure, a high-calorie diet and adequate fluid intake, and bed rest. Patients may receive an analgesic to relieve pleuritic chest pain.

What to do

These interventions aim to increase patient comfort, avoid complications, and speed recovery:

• Maintain a patent airway and adequate oxygenation. Measure ABG levels, especially in hypoxic patients. Administer supplemental oxygen as ordered. Use caution when administering oxygen to patients with underlying COPD.

• Administer antibiotics as ordered and pain medication as needed. Fever and dehydration may require I.V. fluids and electrolyte replacement.

• Maintain adequate nutrition to offset extra calories burned during infection. Ask the dietary department to provide a high-calorie, high-protein diet consisting of soft, easy-to-eat foods. Encourage the patient to eat. Monitor fluid intake and output.

• To control the spread of infection, dispose of secretions properly. Tell the patient to sneeze and cough into a disposable tissue; tape a waxed bag to the side of the bed for used tissues.

• To prevent aspiration during NG tube feedings, elevate the patient's head, check the position of the tube, and administer feedings slowly. Don't give large volumes at one time because this could cause vomiting. If the patient has a tracheostomy or an ET tube, inflate the tube cuff. Keep his head elevated for at least 30 minutes after feeding.

• Be aware that antimicrobial agents used to treat cytomegalovirus, *P. carinii*, and respiratory syncytial virus pneumonia may be hazardous to fetal development. Pregnant health care workers or those attempting conception should minimize exposure to these agents (such as acyclovir, ribavirin, and pentamidine).

• Evaluate the patient. His chest X-rays should be normal and his ABG levels should show PaO_2 of 50 to 60 mm Hg. (See *Teaching the patient with pneumonia*.)

Pneumothorax

In pneumothorax, air or gas accumulates between the parietal and visceral pleurae, causing the lungs to collapse. The amount of air or gas trapped determines the de-

---

Teaching the patient with pneumonia

Teach the patient how to cough and perform deep-breathing exercises to clear secretions.

Prevention pearls

To help prevent pneumonia, urge all postoperative and bedridden patients to perform deep-breathing exercises frequently. Position patients properly to promote full ventilation and drainage of secretions. Also encourage annual influenza and pneumococcal vaccination for high-risk patients, such as those with chronic obstructive pulmonary disease, chronic heart disease, or sickle cell disease.

Furthermore, advise the patient to avoid using antibiotics indiscriminately during minor viral infections. Explain that doing so may result in the colonization of antibiotic-resistant bacteria in the upper airway. If the patient then develops pneumonia, the infecting organisms may require treatment with more toxic antibiotics.

gree of lung collapse. In some cases, venous return to the heart is impeded, causing a life-threatening condition called *tension pneumothorax.*

An open or shut case

Pneumothorax is classified as either traumatic or spontaneous. *Traumatic pneumothorax* may be further classified as open (sucking chest wound) or closed (blunt or penetrating trauma). Note that if an open (penetrating) wound seals itself off, stopping communication between the atmosphere and the pleural space, a closed pneumothorax may result. *Spontaneous pneumothorax,* which is also considered closed, can be further classified as primary (idiopathic) or secondary (related to a specific disease).

What causes it

Traumatic pneumothorax can result from:
- insertion of a central venous pressure line
- thoracic surgery
- thoracentesis or closed pleural biopsy
- penetrating chest injury
- transbronchial biopsy.
   Spontaneous pneumothorax can result from:
- ruptured congenital blebs
- ruptured emphysematous bullae
- tubercular or malignant lesions that erode into the pleural space
- interstitial lung disease, such as eosinophilic granuloma.
   Tension pneumothorax can develop from either traumatic or spontaneous pneumothorax. (See *Understanding tension pneumothorax,* page 176.)

Pathophysiology

The pathophysiology of pneumothorax varies according to classification.

A change in atmosphere

Open pneumothorax results when atmospheric air (positive pressure) flows directly into the pleural cavity (negative pressure). As the air pressure in the pleural cavity becomes positive, the lung collapses on the affected side.

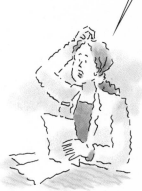

Let's see... Pneumothorax can be either traumatic or spontaneous. Traumatic pneumothorax can be either open or closed. Spontaneous pneumothorax is closed, but it can be classified as primary or secondary.

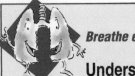

Breathe easy

Understanding tension pneumothorax

In tension pneumothorax, air accumulates intrapleurally and can't escape. Intrapleural pressure rises, collapsing the ipsilateral lung.

Breathe in
On inspiration, the mediastinum shifts toward the unaffected lung, impairing ventilation.

Breathe out
On expiration, the mediastinal shift distorts the vena cava and reduces venous return.

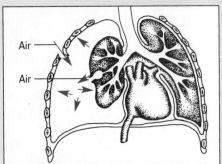

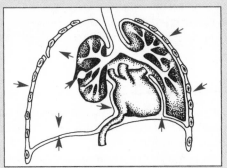

Lung collapse leads to decreased total lung capacity, causing hypoxia.

An inside job

Closed pneumothorax occurs when air enters the pleural space from within the lung. This causes increased pleural pressure, which prevents lung expansion during inspiration. It may be called *traumatic* pneumothorax when blunt chest trauma causes lung tissue to rupture, resulting in air leakage.

Explosive situation

Spontaneous pneumothorax is a type of closed pneumothorax that usually results when a subpleural bleb (a small cystic space) at the surface of the lung ruptures. This rupture causes air leakage into the pleural spaces; then the lung collapses, causing decreased total lung capacity, vital capacity, and lung compliance—leading, in turn, to hypoxia.

What to look for

Spontaneous pneumothorax may not produce symptoms in mild cases, but profound respiratory distress occurs in moderate to severe cases. Weak and rapid pulse, pallor, jugular vein distention, and anxiety indicate tension pneumothorax. In most cases, look for these symptoms:
• sudden, sharp, pleuritic pain
• asymmetrical chest wall movement
• shortness of breath
• cyanosis
• decreased or absent breath sounds over the collapsed lung
• hyperresonance on the affected side
• crackling beneath the skin on palpation (subcutaneous emphysema).

What tests tell you

• Chest X-rays show air in the pleural space and may reveal mediastinal shift.
• If pneumothorax is significant, ABG findings include pH less than 7.35, PaO_2 less than 80 mm Hg, and $PaCO_2$ above 45 mm Hg.

How it's treated

Treatment is conservative for spontaneous pneumothorax in cases where no signs of increased pleural pressure appear, lung collapse is less than 30%, and the patient shows no signs of dyspnea or other indications of physiologic compromise. Such treatment consists of bed rest or activity as tolerated by the patient; careful monitoring of blood pressure, pulse rate, and respirations; and oxygen administration. Some patients may require needle aspiration of the air using a large-bore needle attached to a syringe.

Pressure relief valve

Keep in mind that, when more than 30% of the lung has collapsed, the patient will require a thoracotomy tube to allow air to rise to the top of the intrapleural space. Placed in the second or third intercostal space at the midclavicular line, the tube is then connected to an underwater seal with suction at low pressures.

Proceeding with procedures

Patients experiencing recurrent spontaneous pneumo-
thoraxes will require a thoracotomy and pleurectomy.
These procedures prevent recurrence by causing the
lung to adhere to the parietal pleura. Patients with
traumatic or tension pneumothorax require chest
tube drainage. Traumatic pneumothorax may also
require surgical repair.

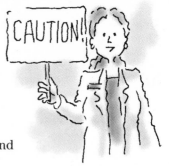

What to do

The following measures aim to prevent complications and
increase patient comfort:
• Watch for pallor, gasping respirations, and sudden chest
pain.
• Carefully monitor vital signs at least every hour for indications of shock, increasing respiratory distress, or mediastinal shift. Listen for breath sounds over both lungs.
Falling blood pressure with rising pulse and respiratory
rates may indicate tension pneumothorax, which can be
fatal if not promptly treated.
• Make the patient as comfortable as possible — a patient
with pneumothorax is usually most comfortable sitting
upright.
• Urge the patient to control coughing and gasping during
thoracotomy.
• After the chest tube is in place, encourage him to cough
and breathe deeply at least once per hour to facilitate lung
expansion.
• In the patient undergoing chest tube drainage, watch for
continuing air leakage (bubbling) in the water-seal chamber. This indicates the lung defect has failed to close and
may require surgery. Also observe for increasing subcutaneous emphysema by checking around the neck or at the
tube insertion site for crackling beneath the skin. If the
patient is on a ventilator, be alert for difficulty in breathing in time with the ventilator as you monitor its gauges
for pressure increases.
• Change dressings around the chest tube insertion site as
needed and as per your facility's policy. Be careful not to
reposition or dislodge the tube. If the tube dislodges, immediately place a petroleum gauze dressing over the
opening to prevent rapid lung collapse.
• Observe the chest tube site for leakage and note the
amount and color of drainage. Walk the patient as ordered

**Memory
jogger**

When your
patient is
undergoing chest
tube drainage, be an
ACE at detecting
these signs of trou-
ble:

Air leaks — continu-
ous bubbling in the
water-seal chamber
may indicate that
the system has a
leak or that the lung
defect has failed to
close

Crackling beneath
the skin at the chest
tube insertion site —
heralds increasing
subcutaneous em-
physema

Erratic breathing —
may indicate impend-
ing tension pneu-
mothorax.

(usually on the first postoperative day) to facilitate deep inspiration and lung expansion.
• Evaluate the patient. Chest X-rays, respiratory rate and depth, and vital signs should be normal. (See *Teaching the patient with pneumothorax.*)

Pulmonary edema

Pulmonary edema is a common complication of cardiac disorders. It's marked by accumulated fluid in the lung's extravascular spaces. It may occur as a chronic condition or develop quickly, rapidly becoming fatal.

What causes it

Pulmonary edema may result from left-sided heart failure caused by:
• arteriosclerosis
• cardiomyopathy
• hypertension
• valvular heart disease.

Pathophysiology

Normally, pulmonary capillary hydrostatic pressure, capillary oncotic pressure, capillary permeability, and lymphatic drainage are in balance. This prevents fluid infiltration to the lungs. When this balance changes, or the lymphatic drainage system is obstructed, pulmonary edema results.

Let the force be with you

If colloid osmotic pressure decreases, the hydrostatic force that regulates intravascular fluids is lost because nothing opposes it. Fluid flows freely into the interstitium and alveoli, impairing gas exchange and leading to pulmonary edema. (See *Understanding pulmonary edema*, page 180.)

What to look for

Signs and symptoms vary with the stage of pulmonary edema.
  In the early stages, look for:
• dyspnea on exertion
• paroxysmal nocturnal dyspnea
• orthopnea

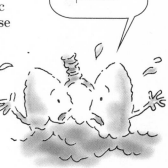

Hey! Who turned down the osmotic pressure?

Breathe easy

Understanding pulmonary edema

In pulmonary edema, diminished function of the left ventricle causes blood to pool there and in the left atrium. Eventually, blood backs up into the pulmonary veins and capillaries.

Increasing capillary hydrostatic pressure pushes fluid into the interstitial spaces and alveoli. The illustrations below show a normal alveolus and the effects of pulmonary edema.

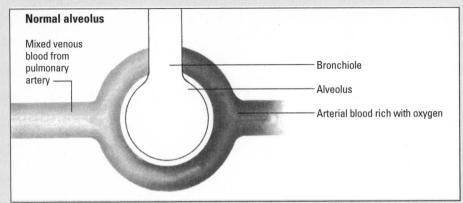

Normal alveolus

Mixed venous blood from pulmonary artery

Bronchiole

Alveolus

Arterial blood rich with oxygen

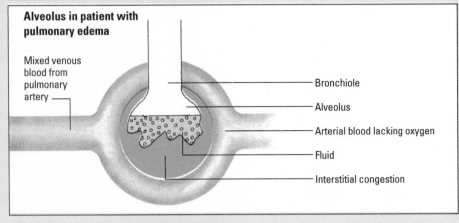

Alveolus in patient with pulmonary edema

Mixed venous blood from pulmonary artery

Bronchiole

Alveolus

Arterial blood lacking oxygen

Fluid

Interstitial congestion

- cough
- mild tachypnea
- dependent crackles
- increased blood pressure
- neck vein distention
- diastolic S_3 gallop
- tachycardia.

As tissue hypoxia and decreased cardiac output occur, you'll see:
- labored, rapid respiration
- more diffuse crackles
- cough producing frothy, bloody sputum
- increased tachycardia
- falling blood pressure
- thready pulse
- arrhythmias
- cold, clammy skin
- diaphoresis
- cyanosis.

What tests tell you

Clinical features of pulmonary edema permit a working diagnosis. These diagnostic tests are used to confirm the disease:
- ABG analysis usually shows hypoxia with variable $Paco_2$, depending on the patient's degree of fatigue. Metabolic acidosis may be revealed.
- Chest X-rays show diffuse haziness of the lung fields and, usually, cardiomegaly and pleural effusion. Sequential chest X-rays show whether thoracostomy was effective in resolving pneumothorax.
- Pulse oximetry may reveal decreasing Sao_2 levels.
- PA catheterization identifies left-sided heart failure and helps rule out ARDS.
- ECG may show previous or current MI.

How it's treated

Treatment of pulmonary edema is directed toward reducing extravascular fluid, improving gas exchange and myocardial function, and correcting the underlying disease if possible. Patients typically receive a high concentration of oxygen delivered by cannula. If arterial oxygen levels remain low, assisted ventilation may be necessary.

Time to dry out

Diuretics are given to mobilize extravascular fluid. Patients may also receive positive inotropic agents to enhance myocardial contractility, pressor agents to enhance contractility and promote vasoconstriction, and arterial vasodilators. Morphine is used to reduce anxiety and dyspnea.

What to do

When caring for a patient with pulmonary edema, consider these interventions:
• Help the patient relax to promote oxygenation, control bronchospasm, and enhance myocardial contractility.
• Reassure the patient, who's likely to be frightened by his inability to breathe normally. Provide emotional support to family members as well.
• Place the patient in high Fowler's position to enhance lung expansion.
• Administer oxygen as ordered.
• Assess the patient's condition frequently and document his responses to treatment. Monitor ABG and pulse oximetry values, oral and I.V. fluid intake, urine output and, in the patient with a PA catheter, pulmonary end-diastolic and pulmonary artery wedge pressures. Check the cardiac monitor often and report changes immediately.
• Watch for complications of such treatments as electrolyte depletion, oxygen therapy, and mechanical ventilation.
• Monitor vital signs every 15 to 30 minutes while administering nitroprusside in dextrose 5% in water by I.V. drip. During use, protect the solution from light by wrapping the bottle or bag with aluminum foil. Discard unused nitroprusside solution after 4 hours. Watch for arrhythmias in a patient receiving digoxin, and for marked respiratory depression in a patient receiving morphine.
• Carefully record the time morphine is given and the amount administered.

Pulmonary embolism and infarction

Pulmonary embolism is an obstruction of the pulmonary arterial bed by a dislodged thrombus or foreign substance. Pulmonary infarction, or lung tissue death from a pulmonary embolus, is sometimes mild and may not produce symptoms. However, when a massive embolism obstructs more than 50% of the pulmonary arterial circulation, it can be rapidly fatal.

What causes it

Pulmonary embolism usually results from dislodged thrombi that originate in the leg veins. Other less common sources of thrombi include the:
- pelvic veins
- renal veins
- hepatic vein
- right side of the heart
- arms.

Pathophysiology

Trauma, clot dissolution, sudden muscle spasm, intravascular pressure changes, or a change in peripheral blood flow can cause the thrombus to loosen or fragmentize.

Prone to wander

The thrombus—now called an *embolus*—floats to the heart's right side and enters the lung through the pulmonary artery. There, the embolus may dissolve, continue to fragmentize, or grow. If the embolus occludes the pulmonary artery, alveoli collapse and atelectasis develops. If the embolus enlarges, it may clog most or all of the pulmonary vessels and cause death.

Rare but serious

In rare cases, the emboli contain air, fat, amniotic fluid, tumor cells, or talc (sometimes found in orally administered drugs that are injected I.V. by addicts). Pulmonary embolism may lead to pulmonary infarction, especially in patients with chronic heart or pulmonary disease.

What to look for

Total occlusion of the main pulmonary artery is rapidly fatal; smaller or fragmented emboli produce symptoms that vary with the size, number, and location of the emboli.

The usual suspects

Common symptoms include:
- dyspnea (usually the first symptom)
- anginal or pleuritic chest pain
- productive cough (sputum may be blood-tinged)
- tachycardia
- low-grade fever.

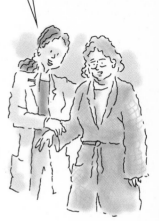

Because thrombi that originate in leg veins are the main cause of pulmonary embolism, remember to encourage your patients to ambulate to prevent thrombus formation.

Least likely candidates

Less common symptoms include:
- massive hemoptysis
- splinting of the chest
- leg edema.

A looming presence

A large embolus may produce:
- crackles and a pleural friction rub audible at the infarction site
- cyanosis, syncope, and distended neck veins
- signs of shock (such as weak, rapid pulse and hypotension)
- signs of hypoxia (such as restlessness)
- a right ventricular S_3 gallop audible at the lower sternum
- increased intensity of the pulmonary component of S_2.

What tests tell you

These test results can help confirm pulmonary embolism or infarction:
- Chest X-ray shows a characteristic wedge-shaped infiltrate suggestive of pulmonary embolism. X-rays may rule out other pulmonary diseases and reveal areas of atelectasis, an elevated diaphragm, pleural effusion, and a prominent pulmonary artery.
- Lung scan shows perfusion defects in areas beyond occluded vessels; a normal lung scan rules out pulmonary embolism.
- Pulmonary angiography is the most definitive test but poses some risk to the patient (such as allergic reaction to the dye, infection at the catheter site, and kidney failure related to difficulty excreting dye). Its use depends on the uncertainty of the diagnosis and the need to avoid unnecessary anticoagulant therapy (treatment of pulmonary embolism) in high-risk patients.
- ECG is inconclusive but helps distinguish pulmonary embolism from MI. In extensive embolism, the ECG may show right axis deviation; right bundle-branch block; tall, peaked P waves; depressed ST segments and T-wave inversions (indicating right heart strain); and supraventricular tachyarrhythmias.
- ABG measurements showing decreased Pa_{O_2} and Pa_{CO_2} are characteristic but don't always occur.

How it's treated

Treatment aims to maintain adequate cardiovascular and pulmonary function as the obstruction resolves and to prevent recurrence. Because most emboli resolve within 10 days, treatment consists of oxygen therapy as needed and anticoagulation with heparin to inhibit new thrombus formation.

Massive means more

Patients with massive pulmonary embolism and shock may require thrombolytic therapy with tissue plasminogen activator or streptokinase to enhance fibrinolysis of the pulmonary emboli and remaining thrombi. Hypotension related to pulmonary emboli may be treated with vasopressors.

Seek the septic source

Treatment for septic emboli requires antibiotic therapy as well as evaluation of the source of infection, particularly in cases of endocarditis. Anticoagulants aren't used to treat septic emboli.

Surgery saved for last

Surgery to interrupt the inferior vena cava is reserved for patients for whom anticoagulants are contraindicated (for example, because of age, recent surgery, or blood dyscrasia) or who have recurrent emboli during anticoagulant therapy. It should be performed only when pulmonary embolism is confirmed by angiography. Surgery consists of vena caval ligation, plication, or insertion of an umbrella filter for blood returning to the heart and lungs. A combination of low-dose heparin and dihydroergotamine (Migranal) may be administered to prevent postoperative venous thromboembolism.

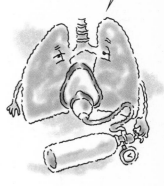

Don't worry. A little oxygen, a little anticoagulant medication, and I should be fine in 10 days or so.

What to do

When caring for a patient with pulmonary embolism, incorporate the following measures into your care plan:
• Give oxygen by nasal cannula or mask.
• Check ABG levels if fresh emboli develop or dyspnea worsens.
• Be prepared to provide equipment for ET intubation and assisted ventilation if breathing is severely compro-

Teaching the patient with pulmonary embolism and infarction

Teach the patient how to use an incentive spirometer to assist in deep breathing. Also, warn him not to cross his legs, which can promote thrombus formation.

Most patients need treatment with an oral anticoagulant (such as warfarin) for 4 to 6 months after a pulmonary embolism. Advise the patient to watch for signs of bleeding from anticoagulants, to take the prescribed medication exactly as ordered, and to avoid taking additional medication (even for headaches or colds) or changing medication dosages without consulting his doctor. Stress the importance of follow-up laboratory tests to monitor anticoagulant therapy. Also encourage family participation in care.

mised. If necessary, prepare to transfer the patient to an ICU per facility policy.

• Administer heparin as ordered through I.V. push or continuous drip.

• Monitor coagulation studies daily and after changes in heparin dosage. Maintain adequate hydration to avoid the risk of hypercoagulability.

• After the patient is stable, encourage him to move about often and assist with isometric and ROM exercises. Check the temperature and color of feet to detect venostasis. Never vigorously massage the patient's legs. Walk the patient as soon as possible after surgery to prevent venostasis.

• Report frequent pleuritic chest pain so that analgesics can be prescribed.

• Evaluate the patient. His vital signs should be within normal limits, and he should show no signs of bleeding after anticoagulant therapy. (See *Teaching the patient with pulmonary embolism and infarction.*)

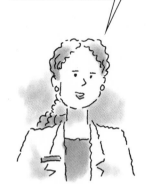

Never vigorously massage a patient's legs. Doing so could dislodge a thrombus.

Tuberculosis

TB is an acute or chronic infection characterized by pulmonary infiltrates and formation of granulomas with caseation, fibrosis, and cavitation. The American Lung Association estimates that active TB afflicts nearly 7 out of every 100,000 people. The prognosis is excellent with correct treatment.

What causes it

Mycobacterium tuberculosis is the major cause of TB. Other strains of mycobacteria may also be involved. Several factors increase the risk of infection, including:

- gastrectomy
- uncontrolled diabetes mellitus
- Hodgkin's disease
- leukemia
- treatment with corticosteroid therapy or immunosuppressant therapy
- silicosis
- human immunodeficiency virus infection.

Pathophysiology

Transmission of TB occurs when an infected person coughs or sneezes, spreading infected droplets. When someone without immunity inhales these droplets, the bacilli are deposited in the lungs.

Send in the troops

The immune system responds by sending leukocytes, which initiate an inflammatory response. After a few days, leukocytes are replaced by macrophages.

Taking prisoners

Bacilli are then ingested by the macrophages and carried off by the lymphatics to the lymph nodes. Then, macrophages that ingest the bacilli fuse to form epithelioid cell tubercles (tiny nodules surrounded by lymphocytes). Within the lesion, caseous necrosis develops and scar tissue encapsulates the tubercle. The organism may be killed in the process.

Dirty bomb

If the tubercles and inflamed nodes rupture, the infection contaminates the surrounding tissue and may spread through the blood and lymphatic circulation to distant sites. This process is called *hematogenous dissemination.*

What to look for

In primary infection, the disease usually doesn't produce symptoms. However, it may produce nonspecific symptoms such as:
- diminished breath sounds and coarse crackles
- fatigue
- weakness
- anorexia
- weight loss
- night sweats
- low-grade fever.

The second time around

If reinfected, the patient may experience:
- cough
- productive mucopurulent sputum
- chest pain.

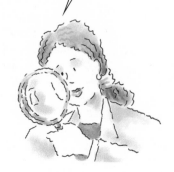

Look for cough, productive mucopurulent sputum, and chest pain in a patient reinfected with TB.

What tests tell you

- Chest X-rays show nodular lesions, patchy infiltrates (many in upper lobes), cavity formation, scar tissue, and calcium deposits. However, they may not distinguish active from inactive TB.
- Tuberculin skin tests detect exposure to TB but don't distinguish the disease from uncomplicated infection. Patients from non–North American countries may test positive for TB by skin test due to the positive antibody titer produced by the bacille Calmette-Guérin live vaccine they received as children.
- Stains and cultures of sputum, cerebrospinal fluid, urine, drainage from abscess, or pleural fluid show heat-sensitive, nonmotile, aerobic, acid-fast bacilli and confirm the diagnosis.

How it's treated

Antitubercular therapy with daily oral doses of isoniazid, rifampin, and pyrazinamide (and sometimes with ethambutol or streptomycin) for at least 6 months usually cures TB. After 2 to 4 weeks, the disease is typically no longer infectious, and the patient can resume his normal lifestyle while continuing to take medication. A patient with atypical mycobacterial disease or drug-resistant TB may require second-line drugs, such as capreomycin, streptomycin, para-aminosalicylic acid, cycloserine, amikacin, and fluoroquinolones.

What to do

Your care will focus on preventing the spread of infection as well as providing supportive care. For example:
• Isolate the infectious patient in a negative-pressure room until he's no longer contagious.
• Be alert for adverse effects of medications. Pyridoxine (vitamin B_6) is sometimes recommended to prevent peripheral neuropathy caused by large doses of isoniazid. If the patient receives ethambutol, watch for optic neuritis; if it develops, discontinue the drug. Observe for hepatitis and purpura in patients receiving rifampin.
• Evaluate the patient. His sputum culture should be negative and secretions should be thin and clear. (See *Teaching the patient with TB*.)

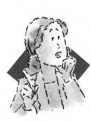

Quick quiz

1. A form of pulmonary edema that leads to ARF and results from increased permeability of the alveolocapillary membrane is:
  A. pleural effusion.
  B. atelectasis.
  C. ARDS.
  D. bronchiectasis.

Answer: C. ARDS is a form of pulmonary edema that leads to ARF and results from increased permeability of the alveolocapillary membrane.

2. Bronchiectasis is:
  A. an intermittent disorder.
  B. a chronic but reversible disorder.
  C. an irreversible disorder.
  D. a seasonal disorder.

Answer: C. Bronchiectasis is an irreversible condition marked by chronic abnormal dilation of bronchi and destruction of bronchial walls.

Teaching the patient with TB

To help prevent the spread of tuberculosis (TB), teach the isolated patient to cough and sneeze into tissues and to dispose of secretions properly. Instruct the patient to wear a mask when he leaves his room. Visitors and personnel should wear high-efficiency particulate air respirator masks when in his room.

Remind the patient to get plenty of rest. Stress the importance of eating balanced meals, and monitor the patient's weight weekly.

Teach the patient the signs of adverse medication effects; warn him to report them immediately. Emphasize the importance of regular follow-up examinations, and tell the patient to watch for recurring TB. Advise persons who have been exposed to infected patients to receive appropriate tests.

3. Dyspnea and anginal or pleuritic chest pain are symptoms of:
    A.   TB.
    B.   COPD.
    C.   bronchiectasis.
    D.   pulmonary embolism.

Answer: D. Dyspnea, usually the first symptom of pulmonary embolism, may be accompanied by anginal or pleuritic chest pain.

4. Pleural effusion can best be defined as:
    A.   a collapsed or airless condition of all or part of the lung.
    B.   a form of pulmonary edema.
    C.   an irreversible condition marked by chronic abnormal dilation of the bronchi and destruction of bronchial walls.
    D.   an excess of fluid in the pleural space.

Answer: D. Pleural effusion is an excess of fluid in the pleural space, which normally contains a small amount of extracellular fluid that lubricates pleural surfaces.

5. In which condition will chest X-rays show air in the pleural space as well as a possible mediastinal shift?
    A.   Pneumothorax
    B.   Pneumonia
    C.   COPD
    D.   ARDS

Answer: A. In pneumothorax, chest X-rays reveal air in the pleural space and possibly a mediastinal shift (shifting of the heart during inspiration and expiration is indicative of tension pneumothorax).

Scoring

☆☆☆ If you answered all five questions correctly, way to go! You can breathe easy about your knowledge of respiratory disorders.

☆☆ If you answered four questions correctly, great! Your understanding of respiratory disorders is circulating well!

☆ If you answered fewer than four questions correctly, no worries! Take a deep breath, oxygenate those tissues, and review the chapter!

Appendices and index

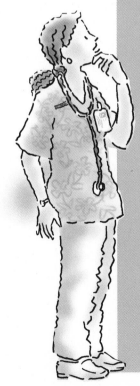

Auscultation findings for common disorders

This chart lists various pulmonary disorders along with their associated auscultation findings. Keep in mind that the patient may not present with every assessment finding listed for each disorder.

Disorder	Abnormal breath sounds
Asbestosis	• High-pitched crackles heard at the end of inspiration • Pleural friction rub
Asthma	• Diminished breath sounds • Musical, high-pitched expiratory polyphonic wheezes • With status asthmaticus, loud and continuous random monophonic wheezes heard, along with prolonged expiration and possible silent chest if severe
Atelectasis	• High-pitched, hollow, tubular bronchial breath sounds, crackles, wheezes • Fine, high-pitched, late inspiratory crackles • Bronchophony • Egophony • Whispered pectoriloquy • Inspiratory:expiratory (I:E) ratio: I>E over empty lung field
Bronchial stenosis	• Loud, continuous, low-pitched, fixed, monophonic wheezes that may disappear when in supine position or turning side to side
Bronchiectasis	• Profuse, low-pitched crackles heard during midinspiration
Chronic bronchitis	• Scanty, low-pitched, early inspiratory crackles not affected by patient's position • Loud, musical, high-pitched, expiratory polyphonic wheezes
Chronic obstructive pulmonary disease	• Diminished, low-pitched breath sounds • Sonorous or sibilant wheezes • Inaudible bronchophony, egophony, and whispered pectoriloquy • Prolonged expiration • Fine inspiratory crackles
Fibrosing alveolitis	• Loud, continuous, high-pitched, sequential wheezes
Interstitial pulmonary fibrosis	• Late inspiratory fine crackles not affected by coughing that may disappear with position change, deep inhalation, or holding of breath • High-pitched bronchial or bronchovesicular breath sounds heard over lower lung regions that are audible through inspiration and expiration • Loud, high-pitched, sequential wheezes of continuous duration • Whispered pectoriloquy

Auscultation findings for common disorders *(continued)*

Disorder	Abnormal breath sounds
Laryngeal spasm	• Stridor heard during inspiration
Pleural effusion	• Absent or diminished low-pitched breath sounds • Occasionally loud bronchial breath sounds • Normal breath sounds on contralateral side • Bronchophony, egophony, and whispered pectoriloquy at upper border of pleural effusion
Pneumonia	• High-pitched, tubular bronchial breath sounds heard over affected area during inspiration and expiration • Bronchophony • Egophony • Whispered pectoriloquy • Late inspiratory crackles not affected by coughing or position changes • I:E ratio 1:1
Pneumothorax	• Absent or diminished low-pitched breath sounds • Inaudible bronchophony, egophony, and whispered pectoriloquy • Normal breath sounds heard on contralateral side
Pulmonary edema	• Inspiratory and expiratory crackles over the posterior lung bases; as pulmonary edema worsens, crackles more profuse and heard during late inspiration • Wheezes
Whooping cough	• Stridor

Glossary

accessory muscles of respiration: muscles involved in labored or forceful breathing; include the sternocleidomastoid, scalene, trapezius, rhomboid, and abdominal muscles

acoustical mismatch: phenomenon in which sounds transmitted through two different media, such as air and tissue, are diminished in intensity or blocked

acute pulmonary hypertension: sudden increased pressure within the pulmonary circulation (above 30 mm Hg systolic and 12 mm Hg diastolic)

acute respiratory distress syndrome (ARDS): respiratory condition characterized by interstitial and alveolar edema and progressive hypoxemia; also known as *shock lung* or *posttraumatic lung*

adventitious sound: abnormal sound superimposed over normal or abnormal breath sounds; usually acquired

alveolar-capillary membrane: cell membrane across which oxygen and carbon dioxide must diffuse in order for respiration to occur

alveolar duct: portion of the airway that's completely lined with alveoli

alveolus: small, saclike lung structure in which oxygen-carbon dioxide exchange occurs

amplitude: magnitude or intensity of a sound or pulsation

anatomic dead space: air remaining in the conducting airways during each breath that isn't involved in oxygen-carbon dioxide exchange

antigen: substance foreign to the body that causes a reaction leading to the formation of antibodies

asbestosis: lung disease caused by prolonged asbestos exposure; characterized by pulmonary inflammation and fibrosis

aspiration: breathing in of foreign materials

asthma: disease characterized by bronchoconstriction, bronchospasm, mucosal edema, and excess mucus production, which lead to obstructed airflow, wheezing, and shortness of breath

atelectasis: incomplete expansion of lung tissue; usually caused by pressure from exudate, fluid, tumor, or an obstructed airway; may involve a lung segment or an entire lobe

attenuation: decrease in the intensity or loudness of a breath sound

auscultation: act of listening to sounds made by the body; usually performed with a stethoscope

axillary fold: one of two anatomic landmarks anterior and posterior to the armpit; formed by the normal contour of the skin over the pectoralis major muscle and the latissimus dorsi muscle

bell: cup-shaped portion of the stethoscope; best suited for listening to low-pitched sounds

binaural headpiece: stethoscope headpiece that supplies sounds to both ears simultaneously

bronchial circulation: movement of oxygenated blood from the aorta or subclavicular artery to the tracheobronchial tree

bronchial gland: any of the glands secreting mucus and serous liquid in the tracheobronchial tree; the main source of bronchial secretions; most prevalent in the medium-sized bronchi

bronchiectasis: irreversible dilation of the bronchi characterized by chronic cough, sputum production, fibrosis, and atelectatic lung tissue surrounding the affected airways

bronchophony: exaggerated voice sound auscultated over the chest wall

bronchospasm: contraction of smooth muscle within airway walls that narrows the airway, reducing airflow

bronchovesicular breath sound: normal breath sound auscultated between the mainstem bronchi and lung periphery; also known as a *transitional breath sound*

capillary hydrostatic pressure: pressure within the capillary system; when elevated, fluid is forced from the capillary system into the interstitium

chronic bronchitis: disease involving inflammation of the bronchial tubes that's characterized by chronic cough and sputum production

chronic obstructive pulmonary disease (COPD): chronic lung disease characterized by obstructed bronchial airflow or exhalation; common types include chronic bronchitis, emphysema, and asthma

cilia: motile, whiplike extensions from cell surfaces, such as columnar epithelial cells that line tracheobronchial tree walls

compliance: ability of an organ or tissue to yield to pressure without disruption; commonly used to describe the distensibility of an air- or fluid-filled organ, such as the heart or lungs

conducting airway: one of the airways beginning at the nose and ending at the terminal bronchioles; responsible for transporting air during breathing but isn't involved in oxygen-carbon dioxide exchange

congestion: abnormal accumulation of fluid or blood in an organ or organ part

consolidation: inflammatory solidification of lung tissue

contralateral: referring to the opposite side or opposing symmetrical structure

cor pulmonale: heart disease caused by pulmonary hypertension secondary to disease of the lung or its blood vessels, resulting in hypertrophy of the right ventricle

crackle: an adventitious lung sound characterized by short, explosive, or popping usually heard during inspiration; described as *coarse* (loud and low in pitch) or *fine* (less intense and high in pitch); formerly known as a *rale*

crepitation: crackling sound resembling the sound made by rubbing hair between two fingers

dampened: diminished sound intensity or amplitude

dependent lung regions: lowest lung regions; the lung bases when the patient is upright

diaphragm: 1. primary muscle of respiration that separates the thoracic and abdominal cavities; 2. part of the stethoscope used to auscultate high-pitched sounds

diffuse: widely distributed; not localized

distribution of ventilation: movement or circulation of air to specific lung regions during breathing

dull percussion note: deadened, or nonresonant, sound heard when a solid organ or dense body part is percussed

duration: length of time in which a breath sound is heard

dynamic airway compression: airway narrowing that occurs during expiration; caused by properties of intrapleural pressure, radial traction exerted by lung parenchyma, and loss of elastic recoil within the lung

dyspnea: difficult or labored breathing; shortness of breath

edema: excessive accumulation of fluid in the body's intercellular tissue spaces

egophony: nasal or bleating voice sound auscultated over the chest wall ("ee" is heard as "ay")

elastic recoil: spontaneous contraction of lung parenchyma during expiration that helps move air out of the lungs

elastic tension: support and traction exerted on the airways because of the natural elastic recoil properties of the surrounding lung parenchyma

epiglottis: small, elastic cartilage attached at the larynx that covers the opening to the trachea during swallowing

equal pressure point: location in the airways where intrapulmonary and intrapleural pressures are equal

exudate: fluid leaking from body cells or tissues

fibrosis: abnormal formation of fibrous connective tissue that ultimately replaces healthy, functional tissue; usually occurs as a reparative or reactive process within an organ or tissue

frequency: pitch of a breath sound; measured in hertz

functional residual capacity (FRC): the volume of gas remaining in the lungs after a normal expiration

gas exchange surface: alveolar capillary surface that's actively involved in diffusing oxygen and carbon dioxide

heart failure: clinical syndrome caused by left- or right-sided heart dysfunction; left heart failure results in pulmonary edema and breathlessness; right heart failure results in liver congestion, increased venous pressure, and peripheral edema

hemidiaphragm: one-half of the diaphragm (either the right or left side)

hila: depressions on the medial lung that form openings through which the bronchi, nerves, and vessels enter and leave

hyperinflation: overinflation of the lung; occurs with air trapping in obstructive lung diseases such as emphysema

hypertrophy: enlargement or overgrowth of an organ caused by an increase in the size of its cells

hypoxemia: abnormally low oxygen tension in arterial blood

hertz (Hz): unit of frequency equivalent to one cycle per second

idiopathic: of unknown cause

impedance matching: similar acoustical characteristics of two organs or types of tissue that allow effective sound transmission

inspiratory-expiratory ratio (I:E ratio): numerical expression of the duration of inspiration in relation to the duration of expiration

intensity: degree of loudness

intercostal muscle: any of the muscles found in between the ribs that helps stabilize and expand or lower the rib cage during ventilation; may be internal or external

interstitial fibrosis: abnormal formation of fibrous tissue that occurs as a reparative or reactive process within the alveolar septa and interstitial areas of the lungs

interstitium: small gap in an organ or a tissue; in lung parenchyma, the space between the alveolar and capillary membranes

intrapleural pressure: relative pressure that occurs in between the pleurae; negative pressure occurs during inspiration; positive pressure occurs during expiration

intrapulmonary pressure: pressure within the lung; negative pressure causes air to flow inward; positive pressure causes air to move outward

laminar airflow: orderly, linear airflow

larynx: cartilaginous organ located between the pharynx and the trachea that houses the vocal cords and allows for voice production

left mainstem bronchus: one of two main branches extending from the trachea that supplies air to the left lung; it leaves the trachea at a sharper angle than the right mainstem bronchus and passes under the aortic arch before entering the lung

left-sided heart failure: inability of the left ventricle to pump blood adequately, causing decreased cardiac output, which leads to pulmonary congestion and edema

left ventricular hypertrophy: enlargement of the left ventricle's myocardium, which can cause reduced or abnormal ventricular function

lobar: referring to or involving any lung lobe

location: site at which a breath can be auscultated

low-pitched wheeze: continuous, low-pitched sound that resembles snoring; previously classified as a *sonorous bronchus* or a *sonorous rale*

macrophage: large, ameboid, mononuclear cell that acts as a defense mechanism against infection; one of three cell types lining the alveoli

mainstem bronchi breath sound: harsh, tubular (hollow) breath sound heard over a mainstem bronchus; also known as *rhonchi*

mast cell: connective tissue cell with an unknown function; drugs, hormones, antigens, and other messenger cells may cause secretory mast cells on the surfaces of large airways to precipitate or control bronchoconstriction

mean airflow velocity: airflow rate within an airway during mid-exhalation

mechanical ventilation: breathing that's assisted or controlled by a machine such as a ventilator

mediastinum: tissue mass that separates the two pleural sacs located between the sternum and the vertebral column and the thoracic inlet and the diaphragm; contains the heart and its vessels, the trachea, esophagus, thymus, lymph nodes, and other organs and tissues

monophonic: having one distinct musical sound or tone; used to describe selected wheezes

mucus: serous, watery liquid secreted by bronchial glands and goblet cells within the airways

normal breath sound: sound auscultated over chest wall areas of a healthy person

oscillation: vibration or fluctuation

parasympathetic nervous system: part of the involuntary nervous system that innervates the internal organs; mediated by the hormone acetylcholine

parenchyma: organ cells that distinguish or determine the primary organ function

perfusion: blood flow to or through an organ or tissue supplied by the blood vessels

pericardial friction rub: characteristic high-pitched friction noise created by inflamed or dry pericardial surfaces rubbing together

pericardium: two-layer fibrous sac that surrounds the heart and the roots of the great vessels

peripheral: toward the outer boundary or perimeter; not central

pharynx: musculomembranous passage between the posterior nares and the larynx and esophagus that serves as a joint conduit for food and air; also known as the *throat*

phonation: production of vocal sounds

pitch: tone's vibration or frequency; measured in cycles per second as sound amplitude; subjectively described as high, medium, or low

pleurae: thin, serous membranes that surround the lungs (visceral pleura) and line the thoracic cavity's inner walls (parietal pleura)

pleural crackle: loud, grating sound caused by inflamed or damaged pleurae

pleural effusion: abnormal accumulation of fluid between visceral and parietal pleurae

pleural friction rub: sound created by friction between the parietal and visceral pleurae surrounding the lungs

pneumonia: inflammation of the lung parenchyma

pneumothorax: accumulation of air within the pleural cavity

polyphonic: having multiple distinct musical sounds or tones; used to describe selected wheezes

positive end-expiratory pressure (PEEP): application of positive pressure to exhalation during mechanical ventilation; used to help prevent expiratory airway collapse and thus improve oxygenation

pressure gradient: difference in pressure between two regions

pulmonary artery: blood vessel leading from the right ventricle to the lungs

pulmonary artery dilation: expansion or stretching of the pulmonary artery beyond its normal dimensions

pulmonary circulation: movement of blood pumped by the right ventricle through the pulmonary capillary beds, where gas exchange occurs, into the pulmonary artery

pulmonary edema: excessive accumulation of fluid within the lung

pulmonary hypertension: increased blood pressure within the pulmonary circulation

pulmonary vein: any of four veins that return oxygenated blood from the lungs to the heart's left atrium

resistance: force that hinders motion; hindrance or impedance

resonance: sound quality produced by percussing structures or cavities that radiate sound vibrations and energy

respiratory cycle: one complete cycle of inspiration and expiration

right mainstem bronchus: one of two main branches extending from the trachea that supplies air to the right lung; a likely landing site for aspirated foreign bodies

right-sided heart failure: inability of the right ventricle to pump adequately, causing enlargement of the liver, distention of neck veins, and peripheral edema

sarcoidosis: granulomatous disease of unknown origin that may cause pulmonary fibrosis

scapula: triangular flat bone that makes up part of the shoulder girdle; also known as the *shoulder blade*

segmental bronchus: airway that branches from a lobar bronchus and conducts air to a lung segment

serous: having a watery consistency

silent chest: absence of breath sounds during auscultation; usually associated with severe bronchospasm and insufficient airflow

status asthmaticus: severe asthma that's resistant to treatment; characterized by respiratory insufficiency or failure, wheezing, and severe dyspnea

sternal border: auscultatory area along and to either side of the sternum

stethoscope: instrument used in auscultation; usually consists of a diaphragm and a bell connected to one or two tubes leading to a binaural headpiece and earpieces

stridor: noisy, high-pitched sound that can usually be heard at a distance from the patient; caused by laryngeal spasm and mucosal swelling, which contract the vocal cords and narrow the airway

subcutaneous emphysema: presence of air or gas in the tissues beneath the skin, resulting in crackling or crepitus when skin is touched

supine: lying on the back

surfactant: active surface agent that decreases surface tension, thereby preventing alveolar collapse; believed to be secreted by type II alveolar cells

sympathetic nervous system: part of the nervous system that innervates the visceral and musculoskeletal system to facilitate smooth muscle relaxation, thereby causing bronchial dilation; mediated primarily by the hormone norepinephrine

terminal respiratory bronchioles: end part of the conducting airways marking the beginning of the respiratory zone

thoracic cavity: space within the rib cage that begins at the clavicle and ends at the diaphragm

thorax: bony structure that encloses the thoracic cavity, protecting the heart, lungs, and great vessels

tracheal breath sound: loud, tubular (hollow) breath sound auscultated over the trachea that's audible during inspiration and expiration

tracheobronchial tree: portion of the airway that begins at the larynx and ends at the terminal bronchioles; also known as the *lower airway*

tubular breath sound: loud, hollow sound characteristically heard over the trachea and mainstem bronchi

turbulence: disturbed or irregular airflow; can be caused by rapid flow rates or variations in air pressures and velocities

type I alveolar cell: one of three cell types that make up the alveoli; covers approximately 95% of the alveolar surface area

type II alveolar cell: one of three cell types that line the alveoli; source of pulmonary surfactant

vagus nerve: parasympathetic nerve that innervates the airways and, when stimulated, causes smooth muscle contraction, cough, and mucus discharge from the bronchial glands

ventilation: movement of air in and out of the lungs

vesicular sounds: term commonly used to describe normal breath sounds auscultated over most of the chest wall

vocal cord: one of two membranous structures in the larynx responsible for phonation

vortex: circular airflow caused by the shearing force of high-velocity airstreams alongside slower airstreams; vortices within the airways are precipitated by airway branching that causes airflow to change direction abruptly

wheeze: continuous, high-pitched sound that has a musical quality; results from bronchospasm

whispered pectoriloquy: high-frequency, whispered voice sound auscultated over consolidated or atelectatic areas

Selected references

ACLS Provider Manual. Dallas: American Heart Association, 2003.

Anatomy & Physiology Made Incredibly Easy, 2nd ed. Philadelphia: Lippincott Williams & Wilkins, 2005.

Assessment Made Incredibly Easy, 2nd ed. Springhouse, Pa.: Springhouse Corp., 2002.

Auscultation Skills: Breath & Heart Sounds, 2nd ed. Springhouse, Pa.: Springhouse Corp., 2002.

Benham, L., et al. "The Development of a Respiratory Assessment Tool," *Nursing Times* 99(23):52-55, June 2003.

Bickley, L.S., and Szilaygi, P.G. *Bates' Guide to Physical Examination and History Taking,* 8th ed. Philadelphia: Lippincott Williams & Wilkins, 2003.

Critical Care Nursing Made Incredibly Easy. Philadelphia: Lippincott Williams & Wilkins, 2004.

Des Jardins, T., and Burton, G. *Clinical Manifestation and Assessment of Respiratory Disease,* 4th ed. St. Louis: Mosby–Year Book, Inc., 2001.

Diseases, 3rd ed., Springhouse, Pa.: Springhouse Corp., 2001.

Finesilver, C. "Pulmonary Assessment: What You Need to Know," *Progress in Cardiovascular Nursing* 18(2):83-92, Spring 2003.

Jarvis, C. *Pocket Companion for Physical Examination and Health Assessment,* 4th ed. Philadelphia: W.B. Saunders Co., 2004.

Medical-Surgical Nursing Made Incredibly Easy. Philadelphia: Lippincott Williams & Wilkins, 2004.

Professional Guide to Diseases, 8th ed. Philadelphia: Lippincott Williams & Wilkins, 2005.

Professional Guide to Signs & Symptoms, 4th ed. Philadelphia: Lippincott Williams & Wilkins, 2003.

West, J.B. *Respiratory Physiology: The Essentials,* 7th ed. Philadelphia: Lippincott Williams & Wilkins, 2004.

Wilkins, R. and Stoller, J. *Egan's Fundamentals of Respiratory Care,* 8th ed. St. Louis: Mosby–Year Book, Inc., 2004.

Whiteman, K., and Kress, T. "Help Me Catch My Breath," *Nursing2003* 33(12): 32hn1, December 2003.

Woodrow, P. "Assessing Respiratory Function in Older People," *Nursing Older People* 14(3):27-28, May 2002.

Woodruff, D. "Protect Your Patient While He's Receiving Mechanical Ventilation," *Nursing2003* 33(7):32hn1-32hn4, July 2003.

Index

i refers to an illustration; t refers to a table.

i refers to an illustration; t refers to a table.

i refers to an illustration; t refers to a table.

i refers to an illustration; t refers to a table.

i refers to an illustration; t refers to a table.

i refers to an illustration; t refers to a table.

Notes

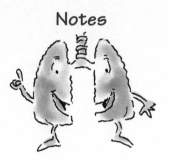

Notes

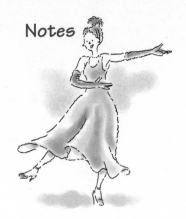

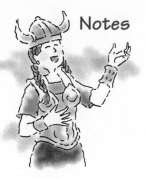

Notes

Notes

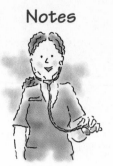

Notes

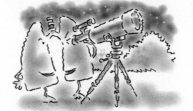

Notes

Notes

Audio CD cues

Track	Sound
1	Tracheal and mainstem bronchi breath sounds
2	Normal breath sounds heard over other chest wall areas
3	Bronchovesicular breath sounds
4	Bronchophony (normal)
5	Egophony (normal)
6	Whispered pectoriloquy
7, 8	Tracheal and mainstem bronchi breath sounds
9	Normal breath sounds (midlung)
10	Normal breath sounds (apex)
11	Normal breath sounds (midlung)
12, 13	Bronchial breath sounds (consolidation)
14, 15	Bronchial breath sounds (atelectasis)
16, 17	Bronchial breath sounds (fibrosis)
18	Bronchophony (consolidation)
19	Bronchophony (normal)
20	Bronchophony (consolidation)
21	Whispered pectoriloquy (atelectasis)
22	Whispered pectoriloquy (normal)
23	Whispered pectoriloquy (atelectasis)
24	Egophony (tumor, pleural effusion)
25	Egophony (normal)
26	Egophony (tumor, pleural effusion)
27	Diminished breath sounds (shallow breathing)
28	Diminished breath sounds (diaphragmatic paralysis)
29	Absent breath sounds (pneumothorax)

Track	Sound
30	Normal breath sounds
31	Absent breath sounds (pneumothorax)
32	Diminished breath sounds (pleural effusion)
33	Normal breath sounds
34	Diminished breath sounds (pleural effusion)
35, 36	Diminished breath sounds (hyperinflated lungs)
37	Diminished breath sounds (obesity)
38	Diminished breath sounds (positive end-expiratory pressure)
39	Coarse crackles
40	Fine crackles
41	Wheezes
42	Low-pitched wheezes
43, 44	Late inspiratory crackles (atelectasis)
45, 46	Late inspiratory crackles (lobar pneumonia)
47, 48	Late inspiratory crackles (interstitial fibrosis)
49, 50	Late inspiratory crackles (left-sided heart failure)
51, 52	Early inspiratory crackles (chronic bronchitis)
53, 54	Early to midinspiratory crackles (bronchiectasis)
55, 56	Pleural crackles
57, 58	Expiratory polyphonic wheezes
59, 60	Fixed monophonic wheezes
61, 62	Sequential inspiratory wheezes
63, 64	Random monophonic wheezes
65, 66	Stridor